Accession no.
36014058

PS 30/4/08

University of
Chester
Warrington Campus

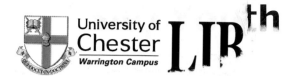

Movement
Performance
for
12-18 year olds

Alan Pearson
and David Hawkins

0193864
LIBRARY
ACC. NO.
36014058
DEPT PS
CLASS No.
613.71 PEA
UNIVERSITY OF CHESTER
WARRINGTON CAMPUS

A & C Black • London

Note

Whilst every effort has been made to ensure that the content of this book is as technically accurate and as sound as possible, neither the authors nor the publishers can accept responsibility for any injury or loss sustained as a result of the use of this material.

Metric to Imperial conversions

1 centimetre (cm)	=	0.394 in
1 metre (m)	=	1.094 yd
1 kilometre (km)	=	1093.6 yd
1 kilogram (kg)	=	2.205 lb

First published 2005 by A&C Black Publishers Ltd
37 Soho Square. London W1D 3QZ
www.acblack.com

Copyright © 2005 by SAQ International Ltd

ISBN 0 7136 7042 8

All rights reserved. No part of this publication may be reproduced in any form or by any means – graphic, electronic or mechanical, including photocopying, recording, taping or information storage and retrieval systems – without the prior permission in writing of the publishers.

Alan Pearson and David Hawkins have asserted their right under the Copyright, Design and Patents Act, 1988 to be identified as the author of this work.

A CIP catalogue record for this book is available from the British Library.

A&C Black uses paper produced with elemental chlorine-free pulp, harvested from managed sustainable forests.

Acknowledgements
Cover photograph courtesy of Imagestate; all other photographs courtesy of SAQ International; illustrations courtesy of Angus Nicol.

Typeset in Photina
Printed and bound in Great Britain
by Biddles Ltd, King's Lynn

The following is a list of trademarks ("the Trademarks") operated internationally by SAQ INTERNATIONAL as at 01/01/2003. Use of the Trademarks is strictly under license. Penalties apply for misuse of the Trademarks. For further information on the Trademarks please write to legal@saqinternational.com.

SAQ®
SAQ® Speed, Agility, Quickness™
SAQ® Programmes™
SAQ® Equipment™
SAQ® Training™
SAQ® Continuum™
SAQ® Accreditation Awards™
Fast Foot® Ladder
Viper Belt™
Jelly Balls™
Micro 'V' Hurdles™
Macro 'V' Hurdles™
Speed Resistor™
Sprint Sled™
Power Harness™
Sonic Chute™
Agility Disc™
Side Strike®
Flexi-cord™
Velocity Builder™
Heel Lifter™
Visual Acuity Ring™ (patent pending)
Peripheral Vision Stick™ (patent pending)
Break Away Belt™ and Tri-Break Away Belt™
Dynamic Flex®
Bunt Bat™ (patent pending)
Side Stepper™
The Curve™ (patent pending)
Swivel Belt™
P-Award™
i-Diploma™

Contents

Acknowledgements

It has taken three years for the SAQ Youth Programme to be accepted as a fundamental tool to assist in the development of youngsters. In that time it has been my good fortune to work with many inspiring and dedicated parents, teachers and coaches nationwide. For all those of you who have embraced the programme and believed in its potential to bring about real change in youngsters, my heartfelt thanks!

This continuing journey would not have been possible without the support of a team of very special people. To Alan, thanks for your vision and inspiration, as without you none of this would be possible. To Sarah, Silvana, Angus, Brian, Marc, Mike, Becky and Danny at SAQ International, a huge thank you for your support, advice and encouragement.

A special mention to a number of superb professionals who have believed in and embraced our work: Geoff Sheldon, Alan Duff, Kim Hazeldine and Sue Odgers, Vanessa Forster, Leigh Marshall, Ian Noble, Simon Brown, Christine Buckley, Jane Mullan and Roger Uttley OBE.

A special mention also to the staff and pupils at Rugby School, to Georgie, Nafalya, Beau, Tim, Toby and Thomas for featuring in the wonderful photographs and to Steve Gilbert for the fantastic graphics. An additional thank you to Dan Barradale, John Steven Chell, David Smith and Wills Robinson for additional photographs.

Finally my thanks to my family, especially Simone and Theresa who continue to inspire me every single day, and my dear cousin Sally, a constant in my life.

David Hawkins
SAQ Training Director – Schools

Both David and myself have had interesting challenges while working with the education departments throughout the UK. We have discovered that grass roots teachers are great to work with and understand the need for new approaches to physical education and learning in today's schools. Unfortunately, we discovered that the few who are in senior positions do not share the same views as the grass roots teachers and are resistant to change and new ideas. Currently the SAQ Programme is being used in over a thousand schools with numbers always growing. Feedback from heads of departments has been not just encouraging, but spectacular. This book is a resource for all those teachers and heads of departments who have provided us with on-going encouragement. A big thank you to you all. Finally, David's perseverance and commitment to the School's Programme has been rock solid. I would like to thank him for this and his on-going strength and vision for future programmes.

Alan Pearson

Introduction

The importance of activity and participation in sport amongst young people has never been more of an issue than at the present time. Newspaper column inches, TV documentaries, government and higher education research and 'frontline' concerns throughout the teaching profession and sports coaching organisations, all point to the facts that youngsters are not active enough, are becoming increasingly obese and are no longer participating in sport.

It is clear, however, that there are considerable benefits in being physically active and in regularly taking part in sport. Health and fitness is developed, educational attainment can be improved, crime rates can be reduced, a sense of pride can be developed and much enjoyment can be experienced.

Over the years there has been a gradual improvement in leisure and sporting facilities and opportunities allowing motivated youngsters to benefit hugely from the support of an army of volunteer coaches and professional sports development officers. However, national statistics (British Heart Foundation) point to the fact that despite this, there is a huge drop in participation once children become teenagers. 42 per cent of males give up physical activity between the ages of 16 and 24. Of greater concern is the fact that 68 per cent of females in the same age range also give up. This trend is not assisted by an imbalance in the reporting of sport by the media. You only have to look at the newspapers to discover that the majority of reports concern male sports and in the event of a female being featured it is often because of looks and physical shape rather than actual performance. Participation by girls in physical education and the appropriateness of curriculum activities has therefore also become a crucial issue.

A joint DfES and DCMS Public Service Agreement target is to enhance the take-up of sporting opportunities by 5–16 year olds. The aim is to increase the percentage of school children in England who spend a minimum of two hours each week on high quality PE and school sport within and beyond the curriculum to 75 per cent by 2006 (www.teachernet.gov.uk). This is a very ambitious target, particularly as a common observation by many secondary school physical education staff and sports coaches is that young people entering into physical activity at the age of 11 do not have the skill levels or fitness of previous generations of children. This makes it difficult to progress through activity-specific experiences at a pace once thought appropriate. Opportunities to revisit many basic movement experiences have to be provided before the specialised skill development desired at this age can proceed. Fortunately, structures are now being put in place to support the delivery of PE in the Primary sector through the successful development of specialist sports colleges and the School Sport Co-ordinators programme (Youth Sport Trust).

Another feature becoming more apparent is the identification, in increasing numbers, of youngsters who have specific learning difficulties: dyslexia, dyspraxia and Attention Deficit Hyperactivity Disorder (ADHD) (Portwood 2003). Research indicates that there is a link between such problems and deficits in motor skills, and a major factor in tackling these problems is to provide structured and sequential movement programmes at all stages of a child's development and to ensure that such work is continued throughout the time spent in education.

It can thus be seen that the provision for PE and sport participation is at present being delivered against a background of major concerns about youngsters' activity levels and the state of their general health. The most important consideration is recognising the stage of development a youngster has reached and then providing the opportunity and correct training to take him or her forward. Motivation is a big factor, together with parent and peer group influence, but probably more influential regarding long-term participation is the success being achieved and the confidence level enjoyed by the youngster.

By coincidence, recent independent research conducted by the Leeds Metropolitan University (Bailey and Morley 2003) in conjunction with SAQ International, indicated that the SAQ Schools Programme had a positive impact not only on pupils but also on the staff in terms of self-esteem and self-confidence. Staff felt confident and empowered by the SAQ Training Programme and appreciated the potential of its inclusion into everyday teaching.

Fundamental movement development

A basic knowledge of starting points is important when considering the further development of a 12-year-old so that strengths and weaknesses can be accurately evaluated.

A process of improving 'good movement', thus enabling physical activity and sport to be accessed more readily, has already been outlined in the *SAQ Junior* book, but a review of the initial developmental process is beneficial.

Movement in children develops from generic movement patterns to increasingly specific and specialised actions (Bailey and Macfadyen 2000).

Initially, by exploring their environments and through trial and error, children experience visual skills, posture/balance, co-ordination and a whole range of motor skills. At the same time awareness of speed and distance develops, along with auditory

and perceptual skills. It is between the ages of two and seven that children lay down the foundations needed to acquire and refine the basic skills of stability, locomotion and manipulation, upon which later abilities such as sporting skills are built.

As well as experience of movement opportunities, changes in growth, i.e. size and proportions of the body, can have major effects upon the ways in which youngsters perform physical skills. During childhood, the head doubles in length, the trunk trebles, the arms quadruple and legs increase fivefold (NCF 1994), making youngsters 'bottom heavy'. This can affect performance of skills, with balance, dexterity, co-ordination and timing of actions all suffering. As children develop at different rates, this would suggest that a focus on the development of fundamental movement skills should remain throughout physical education and sports training experiences, thus maintaining a foundation for all skills learning.

Equally important is when these skills are introduced. There has perhaps been a tendency when introducing activity-specific programmes to focus immediately on the development of manipulation skills without due attention to those skills that should proceed them, i.e. those listed under the stability and locomotion headings.

As previously stated, there is growing evidence that many children do not experience appropriate movement opportunities necessary for the development of basic movement abilities (Walkley et al 1993). It is vital that children experience the full range of the skills listed below (Sugden and Talbot 1998).

Specialised movement development

Having acquired a reasonable level of competence in the basics, children between 7 and 10 years of age (the 'skill hungry years': Maunde 1996, Williams 1996) seek out opportunities to increase the range and quality of their movement.

Stability	Locomotion	Manipulation
Bending	Walking	Throwing
Stretching	Running	Catching
Twisting	Jumping	Kicking
Turning	Hopping	Trapping
Swinging	Skipping	Striking
Inverted supports	Galloping	Volleying
Body rolling	Sliding	Bouncing
Landing/Stopping	Leaping	Ball rolling
Dodging	Climbing	Punting
Balancing		

Table 1. Gallahue and Cleland Donnelly

It has become apparent to those dealing with youngsters who have become involved in sporting activity that there has been a tendency to specialise in skill development too early. There is no doubt that when the focus in a young person's training is a specific set of sports-related skills, the improvement in performance is faster and the results immediate. However, this narrow approach can lead to a number of problems that can have serious consequences on a youngster's future development. Over the long term, the performers may experience overuse injuries, mental stress, boredom, or a delay in developing social relationships, and as a result may even give up before their potential is realised.

Research that has emerged from the former East Germany has confirmed that specialisation should not start before the age of 15 or 16 in most sports. It was found that young children who engaged in a multilateral programme, although improving their performance more slowly, not producing their best performances until 18 or older, achieved a greater consistency in competition, enjoyed a longer athletic life and experienced fewer injuries.

It is not always easy to look to the long term when dealing with a talented performer, especially as everyone involved desires success, but without a constant 'diet' of multi-skills training and a continued focus on the development of basic strength, flexibility, agility, speed and quickness, lack of these physical qualities will never be compensated for by good specialist skills when higher competition is faced in the late teens.

It should be evident therefore that the period between 12 and 18 is a make-or-break one in terms of the transferring of a young person from an enthusiastic participant to a skilled, dedicated and confident sports performer. Engaging youngsters in vigorous, exhilarating and fun learning experiences must be the goal of every recreational session, physical education lesson and sports training session. These sessions will of course be multi-skilled and should always involve co-ordination, movement, decision-making and body awareness.

Thus the focus of this book will be to ensure that a good range of fundamental movement is already in place and, if not, to revisit and continue the process of training it. Once this is present in a youngster's performance it is then possible to move to more complex and sports-specific programmes at the same time as providing appropriate conditioning and fitness work. This is what the SAQ Youth Programme attempts to do.

The above observations indicate the importance of parents, teachers, coaches and educators utilising every possible means to allow youngsters the opportunities to enjoy and participate successfully in physical activity. One of the most effective and successful, stimulating and easy to use methods is SAQ Training.

What is SAQ Training?

Speed

Youngsters enjoy the sensation of running fast. If this youngster's ability is to be developed, a crucial part of the development is the ability to cover ground efficiently and economically over the first few metres and then open the stride length and increase stride frequency to cover a longer distance. Speed means the maximum velocity a youngster can achieve and maintain, usually over a short distance. In Ch. 2 there is a great deal of focus on performing correct running mechanics. This will improve running technique, which in turn will be integrated into all aspects of the youngster's physical activity. The best runners spend little time in contact with the ground.

Agility

Agility is the ability to change direction without the loss of balance, co-ordination, strength, speed and body control. Therefore, to train agility all these areas need to be practised. Agility should not be taken for granted and can be taught to youngsters so that they can become more efficient. Good agility also helps prevent niggling injuries by teaching the muscles how to 'fire' properly and control minute shift in ankle, knee, hip, back, shoulder and neck joints for optimum body alignment. Another very important benefit of agility training with youngsters is that it is long-lasting. Once the muscle memories are programmed they are more likely to remember and repeat the motions.

THE FOUR ELEMENTS OF AGILITY

There are four stages to developing agility:

- Balance
- Co-ordination
- Programmed agility
- Random agility

Although these stages are subtle in difference and often overlap, understanding each stage helps to simplify the teaching and learning process (Smythe 1994).

Balance is the foundation of athleticism. Here the ability to stand, walk and stop while focusing on the centre of gravity, good posture and foot placement can be taught and the feeling of balance retained relatively quickly. Examples include: standing on one leg, standing on a balance beam, walking on a balance beam, standing on an agility disc, walking backwards with your eyes closed and jumping on a mini trampoline and then freezing. It does not take too long to train balance. It requires only a couple of minutes, two or three times a week.

Co-ordination is the goal of mastering simple skills under more difficult stresses. 'It is an activity that involves two or more processes' (Portwood 2003). Co-ordination work is often slow and methodical with an emphasis on correct biomechanics during athletically demanding movements. Training co-ordination can be completed by breaking a skill down into sections then gradually bringing them together again. Co-ordination activities include footwork drills, circuit runs, mirror movements, rhythmic and sequential activities such as bouncing a ball, and jumping. More difficult examples are walking through a ladder while playing catch or performing 'hop, skip and jump'.

The third stage of agility training is called **programmed agility**. Before complex manipulation skills can be learned and many difficult sports movements mastered it is necessary to experience the patterns and sequences of movement, e.g. in learning to play a forehand in tennis it is beneficial to rehearse the 'ready' position – racket back, step to the side, and swing the racket forward sequence – as a 'shadow' without a ball, before a rally is experienced. When the youngsters understand how to replicate the movement programme, they can then give their attention to the speed, flight and direction of the ball. Likewise, in performing dodging movements in a game it is far better to practise a series of different movement patterns in a circuit before having to focus on a whole number of other movement decisions, e.g. where is the target, where are the opponents, when must one move and where are the team-mates?

Programmed agility drills can be conducted at high speeds but must be learned at low, controlled speeds. Examples are zigzag marker spot drills, shuttle runs and 'T' spot drills, all of which involve changing direction along a known standardised pattern. There is no spontaneity of movement involved in this process. Once these types of drills are learned and performed on a regular basis, times and performances will improve and advances in strength, explosion, flexibility and body control will be witnessed. This is true of youngsters of any ability.

The final stage and most difficult to master, prepare for and perform is **random agility**. Here the youngster performs tasks with unknown patterns and unknown demands. Here the teacher/coach can incorporate visual and audible reactive skills so that the youngster has to make split-second decisions with movements based upon the various stimuli. The skill level is now becoming much closer to the 'chaos' experienced in actual game situations. Random agility can be trained by games such as tag, read-and-react ball drills and more specific training such as jumping and landing followed by an immediate, unexpected movement demand from the teacher.

Agility training is challenging, fun and exciting. There exists the opportunity for tremendous variety ensuring that training does not become boring or laborious. Agility is not just for those with elite sporting abilities – try navigating through a busy shopping mall!

Quickness

When a performer accelerates, a great deal of force has to be generated and transferred through the foot to the ground. This action is similar to that of rolling a towel up (the 'leg'), holding one end in your hand and flicking it out to achieve a cracking noise from the other end (the 'foot'). The act of acceleration takes the body from a static position to motion in a fraction of a second. Muscles actually lengthen and then shorten instantaneously – that is an 'eccentric' followed by a 'concentric' contraction. This process is known as the stretch shortening cycle action (SCC).

SAQ Training concentrates on improving the neuro-muscular system that impacts on this process, so that this initial movement – whether lateral, linear or vertical – is automatic, explosive and precise. The reaction time is the time it takes for the brain to receive and respond to a stimulus by sending a message to the muscle causing it to contract. This is what helps a youngster when playing a game to cut right–left–right again and then sprint down the sideline, or the goalkeeper to make a split-second reaction save. With ongoing SAQ Training, the neuro-muscular system is reprogrammed and restrictive mental blocks and thresholds are removed. Consequently messages from the brain have a clear path to the muscles, and the result is an instinctively quicker youngster.

Quickness training begins with 'innervation' (isolated fast contractions of an individual joint), for example repeating the same explosive movement over a short period of time, such as fast feet and line drills. These quick repetitive motions take the body through the gears, moving it in a co-ordinated manner to develop speed. Integrating quickness training throughout the year by using fast feet and reaction-type drills will result in the muscles having increased firing rates. This means that youngsters are capable of faster, more controlled acceleration. The goal is to ensure that your youngsters explode over the first 1–3 metres. Imagine that the firing between the nervous system and the muscles are the gears in a car. The timing, speed and smoothness of the gear change cause the wheels – and thus the car – to accelerate away efficiently, so that the wheels do not spin and the driver does not lose control.

This successful and effective training method can be taught to youngsters through the SAQ Youth Programme.

What is the SAQ Youth Programme?

Multi-directional footwork and body control, hand/eye co-ordination, agility, balance, running and jumping, together with a whole range of manipulation skills such as throwing and catching will contribute greatly to developing fundamental movements and sports skills. These are the keys for youngsters to access and enjoy the numerous physical education and sporting experiences available to them. If these motor skills have been developed through early repetition they become ingrained on the muscle memory and will serve the youngsters for years to come. The brain stores this information and eventually the 'planning' of movements becomes instinctive and reflexive, described by Nicolson and Fawcett (1990) as the 'automatisation of skills'. This can and will bring untold benefits to all participants who continue to lead active lifestyles.

The SAQ Youth Programme is a framework for the development of fundamental motor skills which complements the national PE curriculum activity areas and national governing body teacher/coach

sports coaching structures. The programme is based on sound physiological research and its practical application with youngsters (to date in over 500 UK schools), adults, amateur and elite athletes. Much experience has also been gained from its implementation in the health and fitness industry.

The SAQ Youth Programme resource offers unique programmes which provide simple, well-structured and easy-to-understand activities for youngsters of all abilities and aspirations. It allows parents, teachers/coaches to guarantee a major impact when developing the ability of youngsters to move in a co-ordinated and positive manner.

Continued reference to the skills listed above (table 1) will allow a youngster to be educated as a 'good mover' before and alongside the learning of specialised skills that may involve balls, bats, rackets and sticks. It will ensure that co-ordination, rhythm, balance and timing, factors common to all specialised movements, are constantly revisited as foundations and all youngsters can be challenged but achieve success.

Developing fit and eager movers will go a long way to reversing some of the worrying trends mentioned earlier!

SAQ Youth Continuum

The SAQ Youth Continuum is the sequence and progression of components that make up the SAQ Youth Programme. The elements are:

- **Dynamic Flex** – warm-up on the move

- **Mechanics** – improving the quality of movement by learning how to move

- **Innervation** – increasing the quickness and speed of movement

- **Accumulation of potential** – combining the quality and quickness of movements

- **Explosion** – improving the quickness and control of response

- **Expression of potential** – practical application of all movement skills

- **Warm-down** – returning the body to normal and preparing for the next bout of physical activity.

The Continuum is flexible and allows each element to be used in isolation, e.g. in the early stages or for working with an individual, or it can be used in its entirety when planning a lesson (see Ch. 10). However, the order indicated above does allow for a logical and effective development of fundamental movement.

SAQ Equipment

SAQ Equipment adds variety and stimulus to training session. Drill variations are unlimited and, once mastered, the results achieved can be quite astonishing. Youngsters of all ages and abilities enjoy the challenges presented to them when training with equipment, particularly when introduced into PE lessons and sports training sessions.

When using SAQ Equipment, coaches, trainers and youngsters must be aware of the safety issues involved and of the reduced effectiveness and potentially dangerous consequence of using inappropriate or inferior equipment.

The following pages introduce a variety of SAQ Equipment recommended for use in many of the drills detailed in this book and in other SAQ books.

FAST FOOT LADDERS

These are made of webbing with round, hard plastic rungs spaced about 18 inches apart; they come in sets of two pieces each measuring 15 feet. The pieces can be joined together or used as two separate ladders; they can also be folded over to create different angles for youngsters to perform drills on. Fast Foot Ladders are excellent for improving agility and for the development of explosive fast feet.

JUNIOR, MICRO AND MACRO V HURDLES

These come in three sizes: Junior Hurdles measuring 4 inches, Micro V Hurdles measuring 7 inches and Macro V Hurdles measuring 12 inches in height. They are constructed of a hard plastic and have been specifically designed as a safe freestanding piece of equipment. It is recommended that the hurdles be used in sets of 3–8 to perform the mechanics drills detailed later. They are ideal for practising running mechanics and low-impact plyometrics. They are particularly effective when used to develop lateral movement.

SONIC CHUTE

These are made from webbing (the belt), nylon cord and a lightweight cloth 'chute', the size of which may vary from 5 to 6 feet. The belt has a release mechanism that, when pulled, drops the chute so that the youngsters can explode forwards. Sonic chutes are excellent for developing sprint endurance and have proved very popular with youngsters.

VIPER BELT

This is a resistance belt specially made for high intensity training. It has three stainless steel anchor points where a Flexi-cord can be attached. The Flexi-cord is made from surgical tubing with a specific elongation. The Viper Belt has a safety belt and safety fasteners; it is double stitched and provides a good level of resistance. This piece of equipment is useful for developing explosive speed in all directions.

SIDE-STEPPERS

These are padded ankle straps that are connected together by an adjustable Flexi-cord. They are especially useful for the development of lateral movements.

REACTOR

A rubber ball specifically shaped so that it bounces in unpredictable directions.

OVERSPEED TOW ROPE

This is made up of two belts and a 50-yard nylon cord pulley system. It can be used to provide resistance and is specifically designed for the development of express overspeed and swerve running.

BREAK–AWAY BELT

This is a webbing belt that is connected by Velcro-covered connecting strips. It is good for mirror drills and position-specific marking drills, breaking apart when one youngster gets away from the other. It is also very popular when used in fun games.

STRIDE FREQUENCY CANES

Plastic, 4-foot canes of different colours that are used to mark out stride patterns.

SPRINT SLED

A metal sled with a centre area to accommodate different weights, and a running harness that is attached by webbing straps of 8–20 yards in length.

JELLY BALLS

Round, soft rubber balls filled with a water-based jelly-like substance. They come in different weights from 4 to 18 lb. They differ from the old-fashioned medicine balls because they can be bounced with great force onto hard surfaces.

HAND WEIGHTS

Foam-covered weights of 1.5–2.5lb; they are safe and easy to use both indoors and out.

VISUAL ACUITY RING

A hard plastic ring of approx 30 inches in diameter with 3 or 4 different coloured balls attached to it, all equally distributed around the ring. The ring helps to develop visual acuity and tracking skills when thrown and caught between the youngsters.

PERIPHERAL VISION STICK

The stick is simple but very effective for the training of peripheral vision. It is about 4 feet long with a brightly coloured ball at one end. Once again this is an effective piece of equipment for all youngsters.

BUNT BAT

A 4-foot stick with three coloured balls – one at each end and one in the middle. Working in pairs, youngster 1 holds the bat with two hands while youngster 2 throws a small ball or bean bag for youngster 1 to 'bunt' or fend off. This is effective for all youngsters but particularly so for their hand–eye co-ordination.

AGILITY DISC

An inflatable rubber disc 18 inches across. The discs are multi-purpose but particularly good for proprioceptive and core development work (to strengthen the deep muscles of the trunk). They can be stood on, knelt on, sat on and lain on for the performance of all types of drills.

SIDESTRIKE

A heavy-duty platform with raised angled ends for foot placement. Ends are adjustable to accommodate different-sized athletes, surface is padded to provide protection. A fantastic piece of equipment for explosive footwork development, ideal for goal-keepers, cricketers and tennis players.

How to use this book

This book is intended to assist parents wanting to help their youngsters improve basic movements, teachers wishing to improve the whole range of fundamental movement patterns necessary to access the National PE Curriculum, and sports teacher/coaches who are engaged in the development of specialised skills.

Once familiarity with the SAQ Continuum has been achieved, it will be possible to dip into the various sections of the book and plan lessons/sessions depending on the age, ability and aspirations of the youngsters involved. Tremendous flexibility exists to match time available to performance requirements and the accessibility of equipment.

Where reference is made to Key Stage 3 (KS3) and Key Stage 4 (KS4) in schools, this refers to the age divisions, i.e. KS3 affects youngsters aged 11–14 and KS4 those aged 14–6.

Bearing in mind the research findings of Portwood (2003) for those working with youngsters with co-ordination problems, further practice of many of the basic movements mentioned will be very relevant to this population group (see example session, Ch. 1).

Teachers working with classes of youngsters on a regular basis will be able to use their in-depth knowledge of their performers to create differentiated practices and lesson plans (see example, Ch. 11).

For teachers/coaches working with youngsters in sport, the programme is ideal for Long Term Athletic Development (Balyi) and provides crucial foundation work for multi-skill training and sports-specific development (see Ch. 9). Although young athletes move through similar stages of development regardless of the sport they are involved in, it is up to the coach to recognise individual requirements and provide access to SAQ activities at the appropriate level.

Practices explained

Each practice is provided with an explanation of its aim, appropriate performance area and equipment required and a description of how the youngsters need to perform. There is a 'key teaching point' section which has been designed to help the reader learn the correct movements.

One's expectations of a youngster's performance and what is actually achieved can often be miles apart, so sections on 'what you might see' and 'solutions' have been provided to enable the observer to check and improve the performance.

'Sets and reps' (repetitions) are indicated but these are just suggestions. When planning activity levels, it is *quality* not quantity that is used as the guideline to judge the success of performance.

At the end of each page there is a section that provides variations and progressions that help stimulate the reader to provide new and interesting practices and ensure the drills are appropriate to the needs of each youngster (differentiation). Photographs and graphics are provided to aid understanding and ensure that the practical application of the exercises produces activity that is achievable, simple to organise and exhilarating to experience. Readers should feel free to use their imagination so that the activities meet the needs of the youngsters and the facility and area being used.

Application of the drills and practices to activity-specific situations is covered by way of example lesson sections and sample lesson plans and schemes of work.

Finally Health and Safety issues and recommendations are clearly indicated at the introduction of each part of the Continuum.

Key

The following symbols will be used in the drills throughout the book:

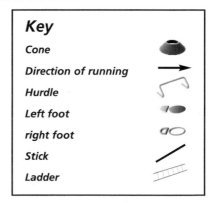

Key	
Cone	
Direction of running	
Hurdle	
Left foot	
right foot	
Stick	
Ladder	

CHAPTER 1 DYNAMIC FLEX

WARM-UP ON THE MOVE

It is widely accepted that before engaging in intense or strenuous exercise the body should be prepared. The warm-up should achieve a change in a number of physiological responses in order that the body can work safely and effectively:

- Increased body temperature, specifically core (deep) muscle temperature

- Increased heart rate and blood flow

- Increased breathing rate

- Increased elasticity of muscular tissues

- An activated neuro-muscular system (the message system that links the brain to the body)

- Increased mental alertness

The warm-up should take a youngster from a rested state to the physiological state required for participation in the lesson/session that is to follow. The warm-up should gradually increase in intensity as the session goes on. It should also be functional in nature so as to prepare the body for the types of movements to be experienced. Additionally, it should be fun and stimulating for the youngsters so as to switch them on mentally.

What is Dynamic Flex?

Although not a standard definition, the following clearly explains what is involved in this method of warming up. 'Dynamic Flex warm-up is a logical system of progressive and functional exercises which gradually warm and stretch muscle groups in preparation for physical activity. Dynamic Flex combines co-ordinated, rhythmic and graceful motions throughout a range of movement (ROM) specific to the activity' (Finney 2004, SAQ International).

Joints are mobilised and muscles synchronised through a natural mixture of contraction and relaxation which also helps stabilise the joints. Muscles work within their range of movement and in a multi-dimensional way similar to what might be experienced in the lesson to follow, i.e. preparation and performance are matched. Because of the progressive and controlled nature of the movement performance, from small movements to larger ones and with controlled speed throughout, the stretch reflex mechanism of muscle contraction is not set off, thus avoiding concerns over muscle damage and soreness. Interestingly, adult sportspeople, both professional and amateur, and junior performers are now reporting, in increasing numbers, a reduction in soft tissue injury and muscle soreness since changing to a Dynamic Flex warm-up programme.

The Dynamic Flex method of warming up is a move away from the traditional method of beginning a PE lesson or sports training session, which has traditionally involved raising the pulse by jogging/running type activities, possibly involving grids and equipment, followed by a series of stretches that focus on the main muscle groups of the body. However, static stretches like these are not the most appropriate when considering games or athletic movements. While static movements are common in Gymnastics and Dance and as such justify their inclusion as preparation for these specific activities, the vast majority of movements experienced by youngsters are dynamic in nature, thus leading to the conclusion that any preparatory activity should be functional and allow for the repeated contraction and stretching of muscle.

The Dynamic Flex warm-up focus should not detract from the need to develop flexibility as a vital component of health, fitness and sports performance. Research is clear that static stretching performs an essential role in improving flexibility. The question is, where is it most appropriately experienced by youngsters in the course of their lessons or training sessions? In a school situation where time is at a premium, some stretching to recover in a cool-down, and as a focus during Dance, Gymnastics and Health Related Fitness Units of Work, will enable youngsters to learn this important feature of maintaining a fit and healthy body.

Youngsters are naturally flexible, and when they enter a PE lesson or a training session they already have an expectation to move; it seems logical therefore to take advantage of this natural exuberance. Using this time for appropriate preparation also addresses immediately the issues mentioned previously: the lack of co-ordination, balance, rhythm and timing observed in youngsters by many teachers/coaches. With the movements that follow in this chapter being practised first from a stationary position, techniques developed carefully, and simple movements practised before the complex, much-needed repetition is given of all the necessary foundations.

A Dynamic Flex warm-up is athletic and stretches muscles in motion. The focus is on motion, not isolated muscles, and as such is of enormous benefit to youngsters as they prepare for what should be an exhilarating experience. The warm-up should not be seen to be 'ballistic' in nature. Ballistic stretching can be defined as 'Bouncing and jerky movements in which one body segment is put in movement by active contraction of a muscle group and the momentum is then arrested by the antagonists (opposing muscle group) at the end of the range of motion. Thus the antagonists are stretched by the ballistic movements of the agonists (prime moving muscles)' (De Vries 1986). The difference between a ballistic and a static stretch can be illustrated using the following: a typical example of a static stretch is an attempt to increase the hip flexion and knee extension range of motion by bending the knee forward from an upright erect posture, keeping the knees extended and attempting to touch the toes with the fingers. The individual is instructed to keep the leg muscles passive and to maintain the stretch position for 15 to 30 seconds. The individual will feel that the range of motion is restricted by the tension that develops in the hamstring muscles. 'One variation of this exercise is to bounce up and down while attempting to touch the toes rather than sustaining one continuous stretch; the bouncing version is called ballistic stretching' (R. M. Enoka 1994).

For those wishing to read further into this subject specific research references are listed at the end of the book.

Health and safety

- Allow good spacing

- Encourage controlled movements in every practice

- Move through the activities in the recommended sequence

- Emphasise care and correct technique when moving backwards

- Discourage youngsters from racing

The warm-up

Using the standard 10 yard x 10 yard grid marked out by marker dots placed at 1 yard intervals for the channels and 2 yard intervals for the length, follow the exercises as described in this chapter. Once foundation exercises are mastered, include variations and also vary the grid. This will help motivate and challenge the youngsters.

SAMPLE DYNAMIC FLEX WARM–UP ROUTINES

A typical warm-up will last between 5 and 10 minutes depending on the age of the youngsters and the length of the lesson/session.

In all warm-ups movements progress from small to larger and from slow to faster. The emphasis throughout should be on the quality and control of each movement. Once basic mechanics are understood these should be constantly reinforced during the warm-up, e.g. good functional arm action and moving on the balls of the feet.

Key stage 3 (11–14 year-olds)

Organisation	Standard Small Space Grid
Time	5 minutes

1. Jogging Forwards and Backwards
2. Jog and Hug
3. Small Skip
4. Wide Skip
5. Single Knee Dead-Leg Lift
6. Knee-Across Skip
7. Lateral Knee-Across Skip
8. Lateral Running
9. Pre-Turn
10. Carioca
11. Hurdle Walk
12. Russian Walk
13. Walking Lunges

14. 3 Steps Jog and 2 Small Jumps
15. Selection of Sprints

Key Stage 4 (14–16 year olds)

Organisation	Standard Small Space Grid (first half)
Time	10 minutes

1. Jogging Forwards and Backwards
2. Jog and Hug
3. Small Skip
4. Wide Skip
5. Single Knee Dead-Leg Lift
6. Knee-Across Skip
7. Lateral Knee-Across Skip
8. Lateral Running with Lateral Arm Movements
9. Side Lunges
10. Pre-Turn
11. Carioca
12. Hamstring Buttock Flicks
13. Hurdle Walk
14. Russian Walk
15. Walking Lunges
16. Repeat again using Dynamic Flex out and zigzag back organisation (see page 33)

Sports-Specific Session (17-year-olds)

Organisation	Split grid
Time	10+ minutes

1. Jogging Forwards and Backwards
2. Ankle Flicks
3. Single Knee Dead-Leg Lift

4. High Knee-Lift Skip
5. Lateral Running
6. Pre-Turn
7. Carioca
8. Side Lunge
9. Walking Lunge
10. Russian Walk

11. Hamstring Walk
12. Lateral Hamstring Buttock Flicks
13. Heel to Inside of Thigh Skip
14. Walking Hamstring
15. Wall Drill – leg out and across body
16. Wall Drill – Linear Leg Forward and Back
17. Wall Drill – Knee Across Body

DRILL JOGGING FORWARDS AND BACKWARDS

Aim
To improve and teach forward and backward movements, the transfer from moving forwards to backwards, body and space awareness.

Area/equipment
Use indoor or outdoor grid 10 yards in length.

Description
Youngster moves forwards and backwards jogging with small steps in a slow, controlled manner.

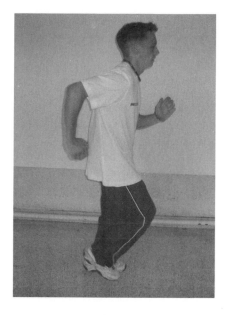

Key teaching points
- Arms to be bent at 90-degree angle
- Work on the balls of the feet
- Before moving backwards, widen base
- Push back hips slightly, chest leaning forward
- Move back glancing to the sides
- Do not turn head round.

What you might see
- Head turned round with a backward lean from waist
- Falling back onto the heels.

Solutions
- Push hips back slightly, leaning slightly forwards
- Maintain an upright posture
- Practise peripheral vision using peripheral vision stick
- Keep on balls of the feet and keep chest forward.

Sets and reps
2 x 10 yards forwards and backwards.
4 reps if moving from a spot.

Variations/progressions
- Rotate core from side to side
- Jockey backwards alternating shoulder turn from side to side.

DRILL ARM ROLL AND JOG

Aim
To improve shoulder mobility, balance and co-ordination; to increase body temperature; to develop positive foot-to-ground contact.

Area/equipment
Use indoor or outdoor grid 10 yards in length. The width of the grid is variable depending on the size of the group.

Description
Youngster covers length of grid by jogging forwards and backwards, rolling the arms from below the waist to above the head. Arms to roll forwards while jogging forwards and backwards while jogging backwards.

Key teaching points
- Arms to be slightly bent
- Keep off the heels
- Maintain an upright posture
- Ensure adequate spacing between youngsters
- Jog slowly backwards and keep aware.

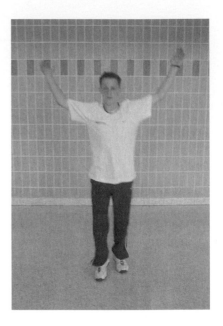

What you might see
- Arms rotated horizontally
- Sinking into the hips.

Solutions
- Youngster to brush arms past ears in a more vertical rotational movement
- Youngster to breathe in, breathe out lightly holding contraction so as to encourage normal breathing.

Sets and reps
2 x 10 yards forwards and backwards.

Variations/progressions
- Alternate arm rotation with one arm rolling forwards while the other rolls backwards
- Perform the drill laterally.

DRILL   *SPOTTY DOGS*

Aim
To improve shoulder and arm mobility, activate core muscles, improve balance and co-ordination and increase body temperature.

Area/equipment
Use indoor or outdoor grid 10 yards in length. The width of the grid is variable depending on the size of the group.

Description
Youngster covers length of grid by moving legs and arms simultaneously in a chopping motion, left leg to left arm, right leg to right arm. Range of movement for the arm is from the side of the body up to the side of the face.

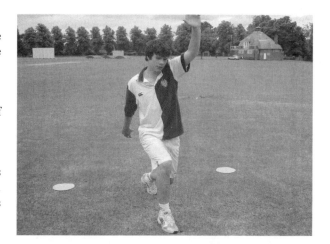

Key teaching points
■ Keep off the heels
■ Arm action is a chop not a punch
■ Land and take off on the balls of the feet
■ Maintain an upright posture
■ Keep the head up.

What you might see
■ Youngster landing flat-footed
■ Jerky, unbalanced movements, poor co-ordination
■ Youngster landing with stiff straight legs.

Solutions
■ Encourage youngster to work on the balls of the feet by encouraging him/her to lean slightly forward
■ Develop a rhythm by getting the youngster to call out 'out, in, out, in' while he/she performs the drill; the calls should coincide with movement of legs and arms
■ Encourage bending at the knees.

Sets and reps
2 x 10 yards forwards.

Variation/progression
Youngster can perform the drill using opposite arms and legs.

DRILL   *JOG AND HUG*

Aim
Improve shoulder and chest mobility, balance and co-ordination and an increase in body temperature.

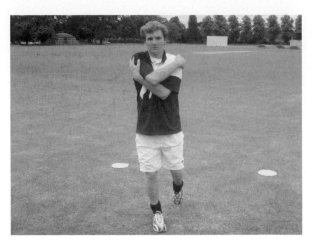

Area/equipment
Use indoor or outdoor grid 10 yards in length. The width of the grid is variable depending on the size of the group.

Description
Youngster covers length of the grid by slowly jogging, bringing his or her arms around the front of the body so that fingers can grip behind the opposite shoulder, alternating the arms over and under.

Key teaching points
■ Slow squeeze
■ Ensure adequate spacing between youngsters
■ Jog on the balls of the feet
■ Upright posture.

What you might see
■ Trunk held too upright
■ Running on the heels.

Solutions
■ Youngster to tilt trunk slightly forward. Drop chin down closer to chest
■ Forward body lean; this will push weight onto the balls of the feet.

Sets and reps
2 x 10 yards forward.

Variation/progression
Squeeze and then rotate the core turning from left to right, right to left.

DRILL   WALKING ON THE BALLS OF THE FEET

Aim
To stretch shins and improve ankle mobility. To improve balance and co-ordination and to increase body temperature.

Area/equipment
Use indoor or outdoor grid 10 yards in length. The width of the grid is variable depending on the size of the group.

Description
Youngster covers length of the grid by walking on the balls of the feet, then returns to the start repeating the drill in a backwards motion while handling the ball.

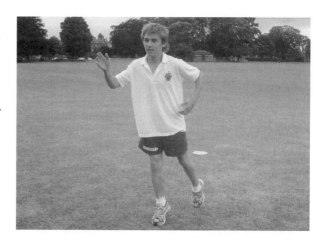

Key teaching points
- Do not walk on the toes
- Keep off the heels
- Maintain correct arm mechanics
- Maintain an upright posture
- Squeeze buttocks together.

What you might see
- Youngster walking on toes
- Legs too far apart.

Solutions
- Youngster to focus on walking on the balls of the feet, keeping head horizontal with the body and leaning slightly forward
- Feet to be shoulder-width apart; use marker dots for spacing if necessary.

Sets and reps
2 x 10 yards, 1 forwards and 1 backwards.

Variation/progression
Perform drill with arms stretched out above head; this will challenge balance and core control.

DRILL ANKLE FLICKS

Aim
To stretch calves and improve ankle mobility, balance, co-ordination and rhythm of movement; to prepare for good foot-to-floor contact; to increase body temperature.

Area/equipment
Use indoor or outdoor grid 10 yards in length. The width of the grid is variable depending on the size of the group.

Description
Youngster covers length of the grid in a skipping motion, where the balls of the feet plant then flick up towards the shin. The youngster should be seen to move in a rhythmic, bouncing manner and returns to the start by repeating the drill backwards.

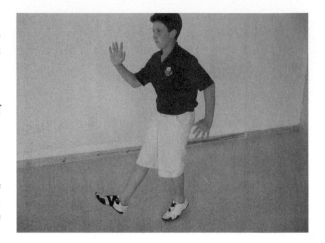

Key teaching points
■ Work off the balls of the feet, not the toes
■ Practise the first few steps on the spot before moving off
■ Maintain correct arm mechanics
■ Maintain an upright posture.

What you might see
■ Poor plantar-dorsiflex range of movement (raising and lowering of the toes)
■ Jerky, unrhythmic movement.

Solutions
■ Youngster to pull toes towards shin on the upward flick
■ Use calls 'up, down' or 'one, two' to help with rhythm.

Sets and reps
2 x 10 yards, 1 forwards and 1 backwards.

Variations/progressions
■ Perform the drill with stop–start variations
■ Perform the drill laterally.

DRILL *SMALL SKIPS*

Aim
To improve lower leg flexibility and ankle mobility; to improve balance, co-ordination and rhythm and to develop positive foot-to-ground contact; to increase body temperature.

Area/equipment
Use indoor and outdoor grid 10 yards in length. The width of the grid is variable depending on the size of the group.

Description
Youngster covers length of the grid in a low skipping motion and returns to the start by repeating the drill backwards.

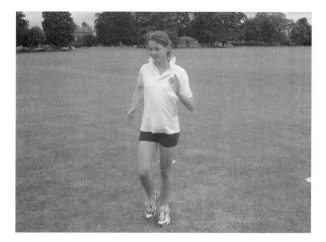

Key teaching points
- Raise knee to an angle of about 45–55 degrees
- Work off the balls of the feet
- Maintain correct arm mechanics
- Maintain an upright posture
- Maintain a good rhythm.

What you might see
- Too high a knee-lift
- Poor rhythm.

Solutions
- Youngster to focus on the knee not coming any higher than the waistband
- Youngster calls 'one, two' or 'up, down' to help with rhythm.

Sets and reps
2 x 10 yards, 1 forwards and 1 backwards.

Variations/progressions
- Perform the drill in a long figure of 8
- Perform the drill laterally.

DRILL *WIDE SKIP*

Aim
To improve hip and ankle mobility, balance, co-ordination and rhythm; to increase body temperature.

Area/equipment
Use indoor or outdoor grid 10 yards in length. The width of the grid is variable depending on the size of the group.

Description
Youngster covers length of the grid by skipping. The feet should remain wider than shoulder-width apart and the knees face outwards at all times. Return to the start by repeating the drill backwards.

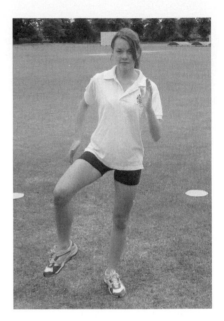

Key teaching points
- Keep off the heels
- Maintain correct arm mechanics
- Maintain an upright posture
- Do not take the thigh above a 90-degree angle.

What you might see
- Landing on flat feet
- Arms and elbows held in too tight to the body.

Solutions
- Youngster to lean slightly forward and focus the eyes on an object 15–20 yards ahead on the floor
- Encourage arm drive; inside of wrist should brush pockets, thumb should come up to side of face.

Sets and reps
2 x 10 yards, 1 forwards and 1 backwards.

Variations/progressions
- Move from forwards to backwards every 3 or 4 skips, facing in the same direction
- Perform drill laterally.

DRILL *KNEE-OUT SKIP*

Aim
To stretch the inner thigh and improve hip mobility; to develop an angled knee drive, balance, co-ordination and rhythm; to increase body temperature.

Area/equipment
Use indoor or outdoor grid 10 yards in length. The width of the grid is variable depending on the size of the group.

Description
Youngster covers length of the grid by skipping. The knee moves from the centre of the body to a position outside the body before returning to the central position. Return to the start by repeating the drill backwards.

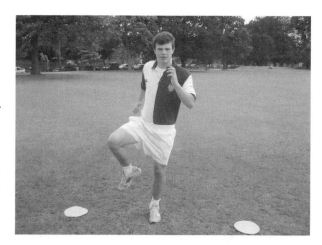

Key teaching points
- Feet start in a linear position and move outwards as the knee is raised
- Work off the balls of the feet
- The knee is to be pushed, not rolled, out and back
- Maintain correct arm mechanics
- The movement should be smooth, not jerky.

What you might see
- Landing on the heel
- Leaning back too far.

Solutions
- Focus on landing on the balls of the feet, trunk leaning forwards
- Keep head slightly dipped towards chest.

Sets and reps
2 x 10 yards, 1 forwards and 1 backwards.

Variations/progressions
- Perform the drill slowly while rotating 360 degrees, knee out every 90 degrees
- Perform the drill laterally.

DRILL SINGLE-KNEE DEAD-LEG LIFT

Aim

To improve buttock flexibility and hip mobility; to isolate the correct 'running cycle' motion for each leg.

Area/equipment

Use indoor or outdoor grid 10 yards in length. The width of the grid is variable depending on the size of the group.

Description

Youngster covers length of the grid by bringing the knee of one leg quickly up to a 90-degree position. The other leg should remain as straight as possible with a very short lift away from the ground throughout the movement. The ratio should be 1 : 4, i.e. 1 lift to every 4 steps. Work one leg on the way down the grid and the other on the return.

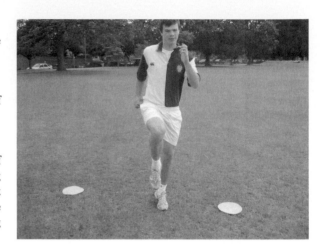

Key teaching points

- Do not raise knees above 90 degrees
- Strike the floor with the ball of the foot
- Keep the foot in a linear position
- Maintain correct running mechanics.

What you might see

- Both knees being lifted
- Stuttering form and rhythm
- Knee-lift angled either out or across the body.

Solutions

- Youngster to focus on one side only. Perform the drill at a walking pace, i.e. walk, lift, walk, lift
- Use marker dots to help rhythm; work on this drill in the mechanics phase
- Perform drill with the arm on the knee-lift side held out in a linear position with the open palm of the hand facing downwards; knee to be brought up to touch the palm of the hand and return to the ground.

Sets and reps

2 x 10 yards, 1 forwards and 1 backwards.

Variation/progression

Vary the lift ratio, e.g. 1 : 2.

DRILL　*HIGH KNEE-LIFT SKIP*

Aim
To improve buttock flexibility and hip mobility; to increase the range of motion (ROM) over a period of time; to develop rhythm; to increase body temperature.

Area/equipment
Use indoor or outdoor grid 10 yards in length. The width of the grid is variable depending on the size of the group.

Description
Youngster covers length of the grid in a high skipping motion and returns to the start by repeating the drill backwards.

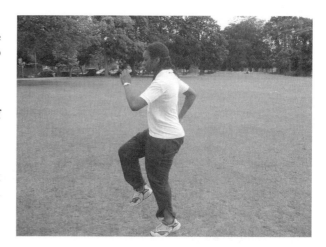

Key teaching points
- Thigh to be taken past 90 degrees
- Work off the balls of the feet
- Maintain a strong core
- Maintain an upright posture
- Control the head by looking forwards at all times
- Maintain correct arm mechanics.

What you might see
- Youngster landing on the heels
- Inconsistency of knee lift (different heights)

Solutions
- Lean forward and focus on the balls of the feet
- Knee to be raised just above waistband; perform drill at walking pace so that the range of movement can be practised.

Sets and reps
2 x 10 yards, 1 forwards and 1 backwards.

Variation/progression
Perform the drill laterally.

DRILL KNEE-ACROSS SKIP

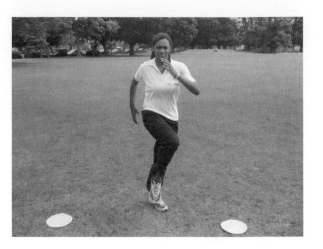

Aim
To improve outer hip flexibility and hip mobility over a period of time; to develop balance and co-ordination; to increase body temperature.

Area/equipment
Use indoor or outdoor grid 10 yards in length. The width of the grid is variable depending on the size of the group.

Description
Youngster covers length of the grid in a skipping motion where the knee comes across the body. Return to the start by repeating the drill backwards.

Key teaching points
- Do not force an increased ROM
- Work off the balls of the feet
- Maintain a strong core
- Maintain an upright posture
- Control the head by looking forwards at all times
- Use the arms primarily for balance.

What you might see
- Too high a knee-lift
- Skipping on heels.

Solutions
- Knee should not go above waistband
- Lean slightly forwards, weight to be transferred onto the balls of the feet.

Sets and reps
2 x 10 yards, 1 forwards and 1 backwards.

Variations/progressions
- 3 forwards, 2 backwards
- Perform the drill laterally.

DRILL   *LATERAL RUNNING*

Aim
To develop economic knee drive, stretch the side of the quadriceps and prepare for an efficient lateral running technique; to increase body temperature.

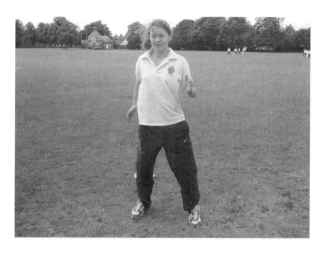

Area/equipment
Use indoor or outdoor grid 10 yards in length. The width of the grid is variable depending on the size of the group.

Description
Youngster covers length of the grid with the left or right shoulder leading, taking short lateral steps, and returns with the opposite shoulder leading.

Key teaching points
- Keep the hips square
- Work off the balls of the feet
- Do not skip
- Do not let the feet cross over
- Maintain an upright posture
- Do not sink into the hips or fold at the waist
- Do not overstride – use short, sharp steps
- Maintain correct arm mechanics.

What you might see
- Feet crossing or being brought together
- Skipping sideways
- No arm movement or arms by the side.

Solutions
- Encourage youngster to focus on working with feet shoulder-width apart. The feet ROM should be just outside to just inside the shoulder using the outside of the foot as the gauge
- Youngster to focus on stepping, not skipping; use marker dots to indicate where feet should be placed in lateral stepping
- Youngster to hold a foam ball in each hand and practise correct arm drive techniques. Youngster to brush the side of their body with the ball and bring the ball up to the side of their face; this will help arm drive.

Sets and reps
2 x 10 yards, 1 leading with the left shoulder and 1 with the right.

Variation/progression
Practise lateral-angled zigzag runs.

DRILL   PRE-TURN

Aim
To prepare the hips for a turning action without committing the whole body; to increase body temperature and improve body control.

Area/equipment
Use indoor or outdoor grid 10 yards in length. The width of the grid is variable depending on the size of the group.

Description
Youngster covers length of the grid by performing a lateral movement, the heel of the back foot is moved to a position almost alongside the lead foot; just before the feet come together, the lead foot is moved away laterally and returns to the start by repeating the drill but leading with the opposite shoulder.

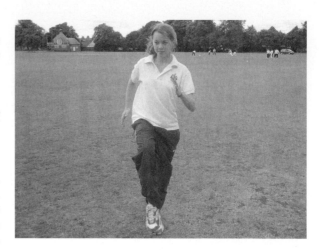

Key teaching points
- The back foot must not cross the lead foot
- Work off the balls of the feet
- Maintain correct arm mechanics
- Maintain an upright posture
- Do not sink into the hips or fold at the waist
- Do not use a high knee-lift, the angle should be no more than 45 degrees.

What you might see
- Crossing of feet
- Leading instead of trailing leg raised and stepping forward
- Hips turned.

Solutions
- Youngster to focus on stepping, not skipping, motion; use marker dots to indicate where feet should be placed in pre-turn stepping
- Use the arm of the leading side to press down on the thigh as a reminder that this leg remains straighter
- Stand tall, head up, breathe in and out then hold contraction.

Sets and reps
- 2 x 10 yards, 1 leading with left shoulder and 1 with the right.

DRILL **CARIOCA**

Aim
To improve hip mobility and speed, which will increase the firing of nerve impulses over a period of time; to develop balance and co-ordination while moving and twisting; to increase body temperature

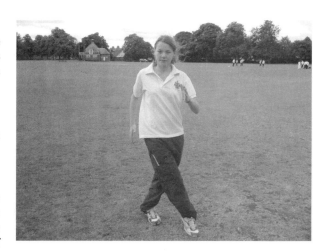

Area/equipment
Use indoor and outdoor grid 10 yards in length. The width of the grid is variable depending on the size of the group.

Description
Youngster covers length of the grid by moving laterally. The rear foot crosses in front of the body and then moves around to the back. Simultaneously, the lead foot does the opposite. The arms also move across the front and back of the body.

Key teaching points
- Start slowly and build up the tempo
- Work off the balls of the feet
- Keep the shoulders square
- Do not force the ROM
- Use the arms primarily for balance.

What you might see
- Sinking into the hips
- Co-ordination problem, i.e. unable to put trailing leg behind front leg;
- Arms swing too quickly or not at all.

Solutions
- Stand tall, head up, breathe in and out and hold contraction
- Practise slowly, go through the drill at walking pace
- Allow the arms to do what comes naturally.

Sets and reps
2 x 10 yards, 1 leading with the left leg and 1 with the right.

Variation/progression
Perform the drill laterally with a partner (mirror drills), i.e. one initiates/leads the movement while the other attempts to follow.

DRILL SIDE LUNGE

Aim
To stretch the inner thighs and gluteals (buttocks); to develop balance and co-ordination; to increase body temperature.

Area/equipment
Use indoor or outdoor grid 10 yards in length. The width of the grid is variable depending on the size of the group.

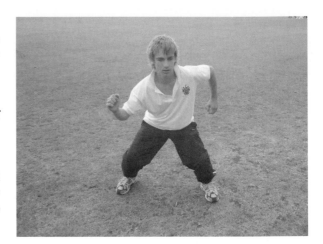

Description
Youngster covers length of the grid by performing lateral lunges, taking a wide lateral step and simultaneously lowering the gluteals towards the ground, and returning to the start with the opposite shoulder leading.

Key teaching points
- Do not bend at the waist or lean forwards
- Try to keep off the heels
- Maintain a strong core and keep upright
- Use the arms primarily for balance.

What you might see
- Youngster leaning forward.

Solutions
- Encourage youngster to keep spine in an upright aligned position by keeping head up and chin held on a horizontal plane.

Sets and reps
2 x 10 yards, 1 leading with the left shoulder and 1 with the right.

Variation/progression
Rotate body after each lunge to face the opposite direction.

DRILL   *HAMSTRING BUTTOCK FLICKS*

Aim
To stretch the front and back of thighs and improve hip mobility; to increase body temperature.

Area/equipment
Use indoor or outdoor grid 10 yards in length. The width of the grid is variable depending on the size of the group.

Description
Youngster covers length of the grid by moving forwards, alternating leg flicks where the heel moves up towards the buttocks, and returns to the start repeating the drill backwards.

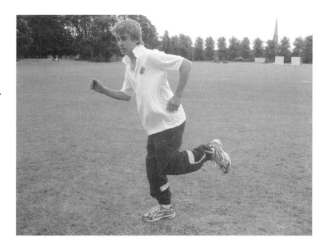

Key teaching points
- Start slowly and build up the tempo
- Work off the balls of the feet
- Maintain an upright posture
- Do not sink into the hips
- Try to develop a rhythm.

What you might see
- Knee raised up towards front of body
- Hands held at the back above the top of the thighs.

Solutions
- Thigh to remain vertical to the ground with movement starting from below the knee; practise the leg flick while standing still, using a wall or a partner for stability; youngster to look down and observe the movement required
- Emphasise to youngster that we move with hands in front not behind our backs.

Sets and reps
2 x 10 yards, 1 forwards and 1 backwards.

Variations/progressions
- Perform the drill as above but flick the heel to the outside of the buttocks
- Perform the drill laterally.

| DRILL | HEEL TO INSIDE OF THIGH SKIP |

Aim

To stretch the hamstrings, groin and gluteals; to improve balance and co-ordination; to increase body temperature.

Area/equipment

Use indoor or outdoor grid 10 yards in length. The width of the grid is variable depending on the size of the group.

Description

Youngster covers length of the grid by skipping with the heel of one leg coming up almost to touch the inside thigh of the opposite leg. He or she should imagine there is a football on a piece of string hanging centrally just below the waist and he or she is trying to kick it with alternate heels. Youngster returns backwards.

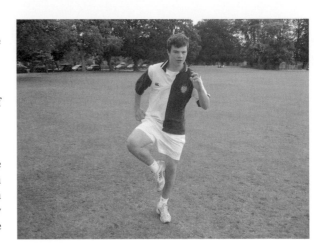

Key teaching points

- Start slowly and build up the tempo
- Work off the balls of the feet
- Maintain an upright posture
- Maintain a strong core throughout
- Use arms for balance.

What you might see

- Confusion between high knee skip and heel to inside thigh skip.

Solutions

- Heel of lifted leg to be directed towards the inside of the groin; heel can touch the inside of the thigh as a cue for correct range of movement.

Sets and reps

2 x 10 yards, 1 forwards and 1 backwards.

Variation/progression

Perform drill with hands on head: this is good for posture.

DRILL — *HURDLE WALK*

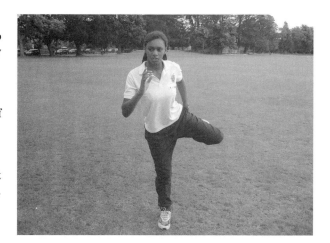

Aim
To stretch inner and outer thighs and to increase ROM. To develop balance and co-ordination and increase body temperature.

Area/equipment
Use indoor or outdoor grid 10 yards in length. The width of the grid is variable depending on the size of the group.

Description
Youngster covers length of the grid by walking in a straight line and lifting alternate legs as if going over high hurdles, and returns to the start repeating the drill backwards.

Key Teaching Points
- Try to keep the body square as the hips rotate
- Feet to be shoulder-width apart
- Work off the balls of the feet
- Maintain an upright posture
- Do not sink into the hips or bend over at the waist
- Imagine that you are actually stepping over a barrier.

What you might see
- The anchored foot is flat while the other leg is raised. This will cause a poor range of movement.

Solutions
- Youngster to focus on working off the ball of the foot that is anchored; encourage youngster to stand with feet shoulder-width apart and rise up off the heels onto the ball of the foot, hold for a second and then return to the starting position, repeating 20–30 times; this will provide kinaesthetic feedback to what it feels like to be on the balls of the feet.

Sets and reps
2 x 10 yards, 1 forwards and 1 backwards.

Variation/progression
Can be performed on the spot.

DRILL   RUSSIAN WALK

Aim
To stretch the back of the thighs, to improve hip mobility and ankle stabilisation; to develop balance and co-ordination and increase body temperature.

Area/equipment
Use indoor or outdoor grid 10 yards in length. The width of the grid is variable depending on the size of the group.

Description
Youngster covers length of the grid by performing a walking march with a high extended step. He or she should imagine that the aim is to scrape the sole of the shoe down the front of a door or a fence. He or she returns to the start by repeating the drill backwards.

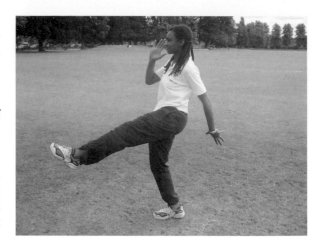

Key teaching points
- Lift the knee before extending the leg
- Work off the balls of the feet
- Try to keep off the heels, particularly of the back foot
- Keep the hips square
- Toes to be pulled towards shin so that they point vertically to the sky.

What you might see
- Toe pointing out horizontally not vertically.

Solutions
- Get youngster to pull the toe towards the shin, and practise the Russian Walk on the spot before walking.

Sets and reps
2 x 10 yards, both forwards.

Variations/progressions
- Perform the drill backwards but do not reverse the leg motion
- Perform the drill laterally.

DRILL *WALKING LUNGE*

Aim
To stretch the front of hips and thighs; to develop balance and co-ordination and increase body temperature.

Area/equipment
Use indoor or outdoor grid 10 yards in length. The width of the grid is variable depending on the size of the group.

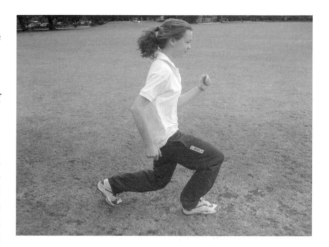

Description
Youngster covers length of the grid by performing a walking lunge. The front leg should be bent with a 90-degree angle at the knee and the thigh in a horizontal position. The back leg should also be at a 90-degree angle but with the knee touching the ground and the thigh in a vertical position. During the lunge the youngster will bring both arms above the head to activate core muscles. He or she returns to the start by repeating the drill backwards.

Key teaching points
- Try to keep the hips square
- Maintain a strong core and keep upright
- Maintain good control
- Persevere with backward lunges – these are difficult to master
- Trunk to be upright.

What you might see
- Poor overall ability to perform the drill properly
- Poor balance and control
- Stride too short causing inability to lunge properly.

Solutions
- Youngster to practise drill slowly on the spot
- Overstriding can cause this; ensure that youngster bends knee at 90-degree angle and that thigh is in the horizontal position; use marker dots to indicate length of lunge
- Focus on knee bend of 90 degrees and thigh horizontal; practise drill slowly on the spot if poor form continues.

Sets and reps
2 x 10 yards, 1 forwards and 1 backwards.

Variations/progressions
- Perform the drill with hand weights
- Perform the drill while catching and passing a ball in the down position
- Alternate arms above the head, one up and one down.

DRILL WALKING HAMSTRING

Aim
To stretch the backs of the thighs.

Area/equipment
Use indoor or outdoor grid 10 yards in length. The width of the grid is variable depending on the size of the group.

Description
Youngster covers length of the grid by extending the lead leg heel first on the ground, rolling onto the ball of the foot and sinking into the hips while keeping the spine in a linear position. He or she walks forwards and repeats on the opposite leg, continuing in this manner alternating the lead leg. Arms may be crossed for comfort.

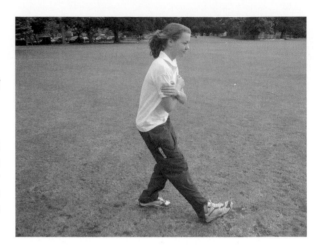

Key teaching points
■ Keep the spine straight
■ Do not bend over
■ Control the head by looking forwards at all times
■ Work at a steady pace, do not rush.

What you might see
■ Head down, leaning forwards
■ Bending at the waist.

Solutions
■ Youngster to keep chin up and focus on something horizontally in line with the eyes
■ Hips to be kept square, trunk and spine must remain in an upright position.

Sets and reps
2 x 10 yards, 1 forwards and 1 backwards.

Variations/progressions
■ Perform on the spot
■ Perform the drill laterally.

DRILL   *3 STEPS JOG AND 2 SMALL JUMPS*

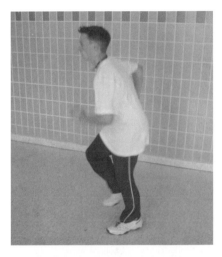

Aim
To improve and develop foot-to-ground contact and correct mechanics on landing after jumping, and jumping after running.

Area/equipment
Use indoor or outdoor grid 10 yards in length. The width of the grid is variable depending on the size of the group.

Description
Youngster covers length of the grid completing sequences of 3 fast steps and 2 low two-footed jumps.

Key teaching points
- Move off the balls of the feet
- Reassert good arm mechanics during the transition from jumps to steps
- Keep jumps low
- Focus on small, fast steps.

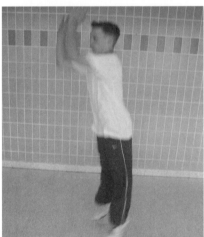

What you might see
- Jerky transition between steps and jumps
- Falling forwards on jump landings.

Solutions
- Slow movements down and reduce sequence to 2 steps, 1 jump
- Maintain an upright posture.

Sets and reps
1 x 10 yards, forwards and backwards.

Variations/progressions
- Youngster should alternate the foot used to take the first step
- Make the small steps lateral or angled in direction
- Return run is backwards.

DRILL WALL DRILL – LEG OUT AND ACROSS BODY

Aim
To increase the ROM in the hip region; to increase body temperature.

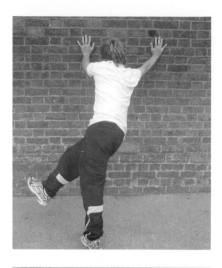

Area/equipment
A wall or fence to lean against.

Description
Youngster faces and leans against a wall or fence at a 20–30 degree angle or is supported by a partner, and swings the leg across the body from one side to the other, repeating on the other leg.

Key teaching points
- Do not force an increased ROM
- Work off the ball of the support foot
- Lean with both hands against the wall/fence
- Keep the hips square
- Do not look down
- Gradually speed up the movement.

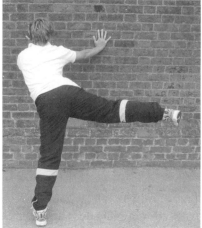

What you might see
- No heel raise off the ground.

Solutions
- Get youngster to focus on leaning forwards and transferring weight onto the ball of the foot while the leg is swung across the body; place a pencil under the heel of the planted foot.

Sets and reps
5–8 on each leg.

Variation/progression
Lean against a partner.

DRILL   WALL DRILL – LINEAR LEG FORWARD/BACK

Aim
To increase the ROM in the hip region. To increase body temperature.

Area/equipment
A wall or fence to lean against.

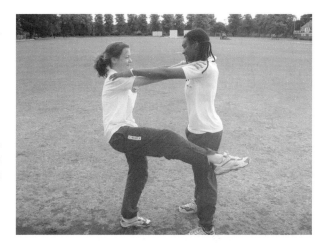

Description
Youngster faces and leans against a wall/fence at an angle of 20–30 degrees, taking the leg back and swinging it forwards in a linear motion along the same plane. Repeat with the other leg.

Key teaching points
- Do not force an increased ROM
- Work off the ball of the support foot
- Lean with both hands against the wall/fence
- Do not look down
- Gradually increase speed.

What you might see
- No heel raise off the ground.

Solutions
- Get youngster to focus on leaning forwards and transferring weight onto the ball of the foot while the leg is swung across the body. Place a pencil under the heel of the planted foot.

Sets and reps
5–8 on each leg.

Variation/progression
Lean against a partner.

DRILL WALL DRILL – KNEE ACROSS BODY

Aim
To increase the ROM in the hip region; to increase body temperature.

Area/equipment
A wall or fence to lean against.

Description
Youngster faces and leans against a wall/fence at an angle of 20–30 degrees, and from a standing position drives one knee upwards and across the body, repeating with the other leg.

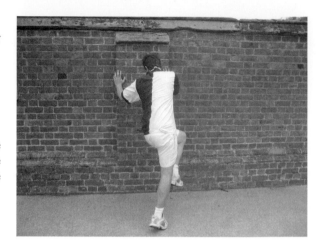

Key teaching points
- Do not force an increased ROM
- Work off the ball of the support foot
- Lean with both hands against the wall/fence
- Keep the hips square
- Do not look down
- Gradually increase speed
- Imagine you are trying to get your knee up and across your body to the opposite pocket.

What you might see
- No heel raise off the ground.

Solutions
- Get youngster to focus on leaning forwards and transferring weight onto the ball of the foot while the leg is swung across the body; place a pencil under the heel of the planted foot.

Sets and reps
5–8 on each leg.

Variation/progression
Lean against a partner.

DRILL   *PAIR DRILL – LATERAL RUNS*

Aim
To develop skills in a more game-specific situation; to stimulate balance, catching and eye–hand co-ordination, and to practise reassertion of the correct mechanics; to increase body temperature.

Area/equipment
Use indoor or outdoor grid 10 yards in length. The width of the grid is variable depending on the size of the group.

Description
Refer to Lateral Running Drill. Youngsters are to face each other 1–1½ feet apart and cover the length of the grid sideways, taking short, lateral steps. Occasionally they can push each other.

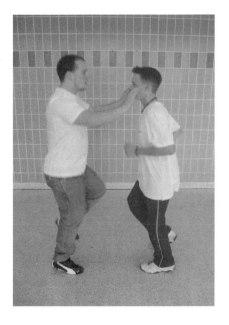

Key teaching points
- Refer to Lateral Running Drill
- When off balance or after being pushed, the focus should be on the reassertion of the correct arm and foot mechanics.

What you might see
- Feet crossing or being brought together
- Skipping sideways
- No arm movement or arms by the side.

Solutions
- Get youngster to focus on working with feet shoulder-width apart; the feet ROM should be from just outside to just inside the shoulder using the outside of the foot as the gauge
- Youngster to focus on stepping not skipping; use marker dots to indicate where feet should be placed in lateral stepping
- Youngster to hold a foam ball in each hand and practise correct arm drive techniques.

Sets and reps
2 x 10 yards, 1 leading with the left leg and 1 with the right.

Variation/progression
Introduce a beanbag and pass hand to hand. Perform runs forwards and backwards; shoulder to shoulder; or facing each other and jockeying forwards and backwards.

DRILL   STANDARD SMALL SPACE GRID

Aim
To dynamically warm-up in a small area.

Area/Equipment
Indoor or outdoor restricted space and marker dots.

Description
Standard 10 yard grid split up into 2 starting and finishing lines, ideal
for organising small squads and groups of youngsters

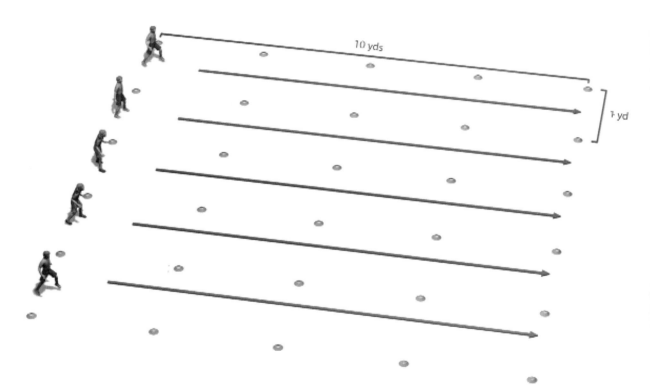

10 yds

1 yd

Figure 1.1 Standard small space grid

DRILL   DYNAMIC FLEX OUT ZIGZAG BACK

Aim
To stimulate and motivate youngsters with a variety of movement patterns.

Area/equipment
Indoor or outdoor grid 10 yards in length with markers placed at 2-yard intervals. The width of the grid is variable depending on the size of the group. Place a line of markers on each side of the grid about 2 yards away with 1 yard between each marker.

Description
Perform Dynamic Flex down the grid with the group splitting around the end markers to return on the outside of the grid. On reaching the markers the youngster should zigzag back through them.

Key teaching points
The timing is crucial – youngsters should be constantly on the move.

Sets and reps
Youngsters can perform the entire Dynamic Flex warm-up in this manner.

Variation/progression
Replace the markers on the outside of the grid with Fast Foot Ladder or hurdles.

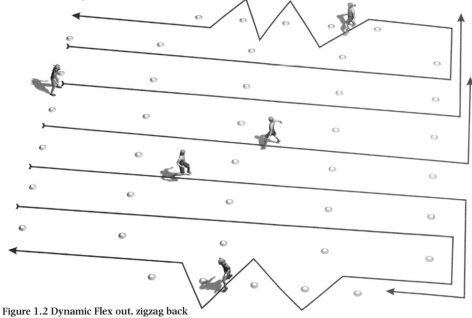

Figure 1.2 Dynamic Flex out, zigzag back

DRILL   SPLIT GRID

Aim
To improve ball control and passing skills.

Area/equipment
Indoor or outdoor grid 10 yards in length with an additional 5 yards on the end (use different coloured markers). The width of the grid is variable depending on the size of the group. Place a ball for each youngster who will have just completed his or her Dynamic Flex drill.

Description
Perform Dynamic Flex down the grid over the first 10 yards; on reaching the additional 5-yard area perform beanbag or ball skills up and back over it, i.e. catching and juggling (manipulation skills). On completing the skills, pass the beanbag or ball to the youngster coming on, who will have just completed his or her Dynamic Flex drill.

Key teaching points
■ The timing is crucial – youngsters should be constantly on the move
■ Youngsters should communicate with one another, e.g. when passing the ball.

Sets and reps
The entire Dynamic Flex warm-up can be performed in this manner.

Variation/progression
Vary the manipulation skills and the objects passed between the youngsters.

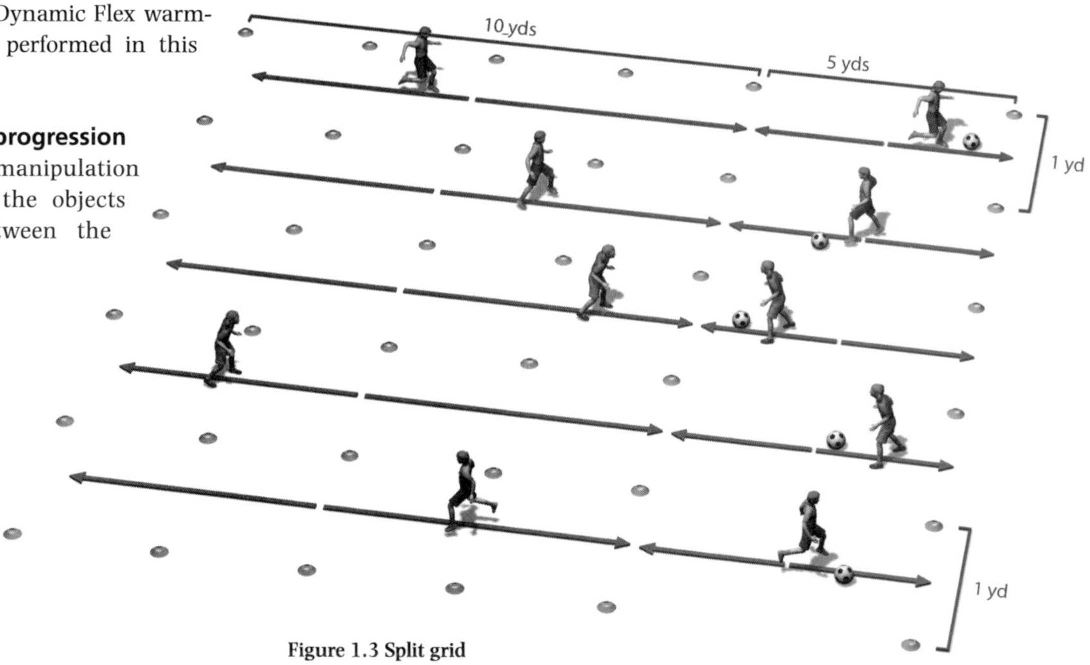

Figure 1.3 Split grid

Additional Grid Variations

Aim

To warm up with Dynamic Flex using various grids to help motivate and stimulate.

Area/equipment

Indoor or outdoor space, various marker dots.

GRID ON-THE-SPOT DYNAMIC FLEX

Description

Mark out a grid with marker dots 2 yards apart. Drills are performed on the spot within the space provided.

Variation/progression

Additional movements can be introduced after each drill to get people to move to a different spot.

GRID CIRCLE GRID

Description

Mark out a grid with an outer circle of markets 15 yards in diameter and a centre circle of markers 5 yards in diameter. Perform drills around the outside of the circle both forwards and backwards. Then, for certain drills such as the Hamstring Walk, the youngsters move inwards and outwards to and from the centre circle.

Variations/progressions

Introduce manipulation skills.

Increase size of circles depending on size of group.

GRID STAR GRID

Description

Use marker dots to mark out an eight-point star measuring 5 yards from the outside point to the inner circle. Perform drills from the outside point of the star to the inside point, then work in reverse.

Variation/progression

Introduce manipulation skills.

GRID ZIGZAG GRID

Description

Mark out a grid using markers 1 yard apart forming 1-yard wide channels, and every 2 yards along move the markers 1 yard sideways forming a zigzag. Perform drills down the channel following the zigzag pattern.

Variation/progression

Introduce manipulation skills.

DRILL   COMBINATION WARM-UP

Aim
To combine Dynamic Flex exercises, mechanics of movement, fast feet and agility in a warm-up that can be used when limited for time.

Area/equipment
Use indoor or outdoor area; set out 1 area for the Dynamic Flex, and a second area for mechanics, fast feet and agility work. Use hurdles, ladders, cones and poles.

Description
First start with initial warm-up using 8–10 of the first Dynamic Flex drills, then move over and perform 2–3 minutes of multi-movement within the grid containing the ladder, hurdles, cones etc. (combination drills), (see fig. 1.4). Move back to the Dynamic Flex grid and perform some more Dynamic Flex exercises. After 3–4 minutes return to the circuit and perform more combination drills. Finish off with some more Dynamic Flex drills then move on to the next activity.

Key teaching points
■ Ensure correct technique is used during Dynamic Flex
■ Correct form and mechanics to be used throughout combination drills
■ Do not sacrifice quality for speed or allow poor movement.

Sets and reps
15–20-minute warm-up including 3 sections of Dynamic Flex and 2 combination movement circuits.

Variations/progressions
■ Vary drills on ladders and hurdles
■ Change and vary the set out of the circuit (see fig. 1.4)

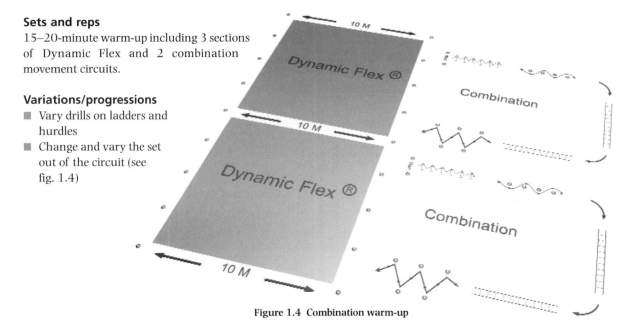

Figure 1.4 Combination warm-up

One of the most damaging assumptions made by those working with youngsters is that running and moving correctly is something that occurs naturally through play. Talented youngsters who make movement such as running and dodging look easy are apparent in every lesson and sporting club, but a real cause for concern is that increasingly teachers and coaches are reporting that these youngsters are in the minority. To neglect the quality of even simple, 'natural' movements in PE lessons and training sessions is to ignore the potential in all youngsters.

How often are comments heard about youngsters regarding their poor running style i.e. 'too slow; flat-footed; runs on the heels; flaps the arms; poorly co-ordinated'? All youngsters, whatever their age, can improve their ability to move, accelerate, dodge, twist and turn by practising and applying the correct movement mechanics.

In this section there will be a focus on arm mechanics, running form, acceleration and deceleration, lift mechanics, posture, lateral and backward movement, jumping, and twisting and turning. Once again co-ordination, rhythm, balance and timing are factors that are constantly revisited and developed. When these techniques have been learned they should be repeated and reinforced in every activity experienced, from the movements found in the Dynamic Flex warm-up, to all remaining activities and drills covered in the Continuum, and to all sports-specific skills that are subsequently taught. They will form solid foundations on which sports-specific movements, e.g. 'jockeying' in soccer, moving backwards in netball and moving sideways in tennis, can be developed.

Once the drills are introduced in isolation it is important to then put them into the context of the activity, e.g. if linear running is the focus, once practised and improved, the practices can be used before a ball is caught and then after to develop 'passing and moving' in a game situation.

The movement checklist that follows sets out the key points that need to be taught when assisting youngsters to start running, accelerate, maintain a fast stride pattern, decelerate, run sideways, turn and jump.

Arm mechanics

- Elbows should be held at 90 degrees

- Hands and shoulders should be relaxed

- The insides of the wrists should brush against the pockets

- The hands should move from the buttock cheeks to the chest or head

Lift mechanics

Teaching or coaching youngsters to get their knees up high, particularly in the first few yards of the acceleration phase, only makes them slower. Using high knee-lift during the acceleration phase has the negative effect of minimising force development; therefore not enough power is produced to propel the body forward in an explosive action. During the first few yards of acceleration short, sharp steps are required. These steps generate a high degree of force which takes the body from a stationary position into the first controlled explosive steps.

The first phases of acceleration and reacceleration for all movement patterns are crucial. Look and listen for the following in a youngster's initial acceleration strides:

- 45-degree knee-lift

- Foot-to-floor contact with the ball of the foot

- Front of the foot staying in a linear position

- Knees coming up in a vertical line

- Foot-to-floor contact making a tapping noise, not a thud or slap

- The foot and knee should not splay in or out, or power will not be transferred correctly

- Keeping off the heels

- On the lift, the foot should transfer from pointing slightly down to pointing slightly up.

Posture

Posture is a crucial part of all movements required for activity including sprinting, jumping and turning. The spine should be kept as straight as possible at all times. This means that a youngster who in the course of play has jumped into the air, and then has to run into space, needs to transfer to the correct running form as quickly as possible. Running with a straight spine does not mean running bolt upright; you can keep your spine straight while leaning slightly forward. What should be avoided is youngsters running while sinking into their hips, which looks like being folded up in the middle, or sinking too deep when landing after a jump because this prevents instant, effective transfer of power. Some youngsters have a tendency to move too many parts of their body all at the same time when trying to run. This causes instability, inadequate use of energy and poor transfer of power, therefore the ability to move efficiently is severely restricted. Core control will help stabilise the youngsters' movement and is therefore another important factor in developing and utilising a strong posture. Core development and maintenance for youngsters is very important. A simple rule prior to and throughout the performing of all the drills in this book is as follows: engage your core muscles by simply breathing in, breathing out and then breathing in again; try to maintain this feeling throughout the exercise, not forgetting to breathe normally! This will help prevent your pelvic wall from moving around causing a loss of power, and will also protect the lower back, hamstrings and girdle area from injury.

Mechanics for deceleration

The ability of a youngster to stop quickly, change direction and accelerate away when dodging and sidestepping, e.g. while playing 'tag', can be practised. Do not leave it to chance, include it in your sessions

- Posture – lean back, this alters the angle of the spine and hips which control foot placement. Foot contact with the ground will now transfer to the heel, which acts like a brake.

- Fire arms – by firing the arms quickly, the energy produced will increase the frequency of heel contact to the ground. Think of it like pressing harder on the brakes in a car.

The running techniques described in this chapter cover basic mechanics for youngsters where running, jumping and turning are all important parts of the movement and are developed through the use of hurdles, stride frequency canes and running technique drills.

Mechanics for change of direction including lateral and turning movements

LATERAL SIDESTEP

Do not use a wide stance as this will decrease the potential for power generation as you attempt to push off and away. Do not pull with the leading foot but rather push off the back foot. Imagine that your car has broken down and that you need to move it to a service station – would you pull it? No, you would push it. Ensure that a strong arm drive is used at all times but particularly during the push-off phase.

MAKING A 180–DEGREE TURN – THE DROP STEP

Most youngsters use too many movements to make a 180-degree turn. Many jump up on the spot first then take 3 or 4 steps to make the turn; others will jump up and perform the turn in the air with a complete lack of control. When practised, the drop step turn looks seamless and is far quicker.

For a right shoulder turn, the youngsters start by opening up the right groin and simultaneously transferring the weight onto the left foot. The right foot is raised slightly off the ground, and using a swinging action, is moved around to the right to face the opposite direction. The right foot is planted and the youngsters drive/push off the left foot remembering to use a strong arm drive. Do not overstretch on the turn. Youngsters may find it helpful initially to tell themselves to 'turn and go'. With practice, youngsters will develop an efficient and economic seamless turn.

Mechanics for jumping

- Both elbows should be held at 90 degrees

- Hands should be moved from buttock cheeks to above the head, both at the same time

- Jump from the balls of the feet

- Land on the balls of the feet

- Trunk to be kept tall and hips slightly leaning forwards

- On landing, do not sink into the hips, use slight knee bend.

Health and safety

- Allow 'eyes down' runs until a basic level of proficiency is achieved to avoid youngsters tripping

- Allow one runner to clear at least 3 hurdles before the next runner goes

- Fallen hurdles should be re-positioned immediately facing the correct way

- Create clear working grids to avoid collisions

- Monitor quantities of effort to allow adequate recovery between repetitions

Observing quality movement checklist for youths

RUNNING – STARTING POSITION

Correct	Incorrect	Solution
Feet position ■ Shoulder-width apart ■ On the ball ■ Straight line	■ Too wide ■ Too close ■ On the toes ■ On the heels ■ Weight outside or inside ■ Pointing in ■ Splayed out	■ Use chalk marks or marker spots on the surface to indicate best position ■ Slight lean forward on the ball of the foot ■ Position feet in a straight line ■ Heels off the ground ■ Use straight lines to position feet so they point straight forward ■ Use chalk to mark around the foot on hard surfaces and stand in the outline to ensure correct positioning
Arms ■ Held ready 90 degrees at elbow ■ One forward, one back ■ Relaxed (see Diagram Check 2)	■ Arms by the side ■ Shoulders shrugged with arms too high ■ Tight and restricted	■ Provide constant feedback on arm technique ■ Practise holding arms in correct position, then accelerate arms as if starting to run ■ Loop string/elastic band around index finger and thumb and point of elbow to hold correct position of 90 degrees
Hips ■ Need to be high – tall – slightly forward	■ Sunk ■ Twisted	■ Head to be held tall and upright. ■ Stomach to be held in; focus on keeping the hips held high and lean slightly forward to the running direction ■ Keep chin off chest ■ Focus on good linear body position
Head position ■ Held high ■ Eyes forward	■ Held down, turned ■ Looking up	■ Imagine you are looking over a fence that comes up to your nose ■ Pick an object in the distance and focus on it

RUNNING – ACCELERATION PHASE

Correct	Incorrect	Solution
Hand ■ Fingertips gently touching thumb tip	■ Soft (most common) ■ Droopy ■ Tightly closed	■ Hold post-it note or something similar between index finger and thumb
Arm action ■ Fast ■ 90 degree angle at elbow ■ Hand above shoulder ■ One forward, one back behind hips	■ Slow to medium	■ Use short, sharp sets of on-the-spot fast arm bursts ■ Use light hand weights for 8–9 seconds then perform contrast arm drives as quickly as possible afterwards
Arm drive ■ Chin to waist ■ Wrist or hand firm	■ Arms across body ■ Forearm chop ■ At the side ■ Held in stiff, angled position	■ Partner arm drive drills ■ Brush the inside of the wrist against waistband, then touch thumb to chin ■ Loop large elastic bands round index finger and thumb and point of elbow, then perform arm drives ■ Perform Arm Drive Drill in front of mirror for feedback
Head ■ Held high ■ Keep up ■ Eyes forward	■ Held down ■ Turned ■ Looking up ■ Rocking from side to side	■ Imagine you are looking over a fence that comes up to your nose ■ Pick an object in the distance and focus on it
Body position – Trunk ■ Tall ■ Strong	■ Sunk ■ Soft ■ Bent	■ Hold head up, stomach in, hips high, slightly forward and square
Foot action ■ Active – plantar flex (toe down) ■ Dorsiflex (toe up)	■ Flat ■ Heel first to touch ground ■ Inactive plantar (toe down)/dorsiflex (toe up)	■ Focus on balls of feet ■ Remove built-up heeled shoes ■ Practise plantar/dorsiflex skip ■ Ensure there is a slight forward body lean ■ Keep head up; do not sink into the hips

RUNNING – ACCELERATION PHASE (continued)

Correct	Incorrect	Solution
Heel ■ Raised	■ Down, contacting ground first	■ Focus on balls of feet ■ Remove built-up heeled shoes ■ Tape up cloth or paper into a small ball, slightly larger than a marble. Place in shoe under heels
Hips ■ Tall ■ Square ■ Firm ■ Still	■ Bent ■ Sunk ■ Turned	■ Hold head tall and upright ■ Hold stomach in, focus on keeping the hips square to the running direction ■ Practise Buttock Bounces (see page 53).
Knees ■ Linear ■ Below waist ■ Foot just off ground ■ Drive forwards	■ Across body ■ Splayed ■ Too high with foot too high off ground	■ Practise Dead-Leg Run (see page 55). ■ Teacher/coach to place hands above where knees should go; practise bringing the knees up to the hand by running on the spot ■ Use coloured tape, stick from above to below the knee in a straight line, either on skin or clothing; now tape across the centre of the knee cap; perform on-the-spot running drills in front of mirror, focusing on keeping the coloured tape in a straight line
Relaxation ■ Relaxed ■ Calm ■ Comfortable	■ Tense ■ Too loose ■ Distracted	■ Imagine accelerating quickly with power and grace, but being calm and relaxed ■ Breathing should be controlled

RUNNING – AFTER ACCELERATION (PLANING–OUT PHASE)

Correct	Incorrect	Solution
Stride length ■ Medium for individual	■ Too long ■ Too short ■ Erratic	■ Use marker spots or stride frequency canes to mark out correct distances of stride length
Stride frequency ■ Balanced for individual	■ Too quick ■ Too slow	■ Use marker spots or stride frequency canes to mark out correct distances of stride length so that frequency can be determined
Arm action ■ Fast ■ 90 degree angle at elbow ■ Hand above shoulder, behind hips	■ Slow to medium	■ Use short, sharp sets of on-the-spot fast arm bursts ■ Use light hand weights for 8–9 seconds then perform contrast arm drives as quickly as possible afterwards
Arm drive ■ Chin to waist ■ Wrist or hand firm	■ Arms across body ■ Forearm chop ■ At the side ■ Held in stiff, angled position	■ Brush the inside of the wrist against waistband, then touch thumb to chin ■ Loop large elastic bands round index finger and thumb and point of elbow, then perform arm drives ■ Perform Arm Drive Drill in front of mirror for feedback ■ Perform Buttock Bounces (see page 53)
Head ■ Held high, kept up ■ Eyes forward	■ Held down ■ Turned ■ Looking up ■ Rocking from side to side	■ Imagine you are looking over a fence that comes up to your nose ■ Pick an object in the distance and focus on it
Body position – Trunk ■ Tall ■ Strong	■ Sunk ■ Soft ■ Bent	■ Head up; hold stomach in, hips high, slightly forward and square

RUNNING – AFTER ACCELERATION (PLANING–OUT PHASE) (continued)

Correct	Incorrect	Solution
Foot action ▪ Active – plantar flex (toe down) ▪ Dorsiflex (toe up)	▪ Flat ▪ Heel first to touch ground ▪ Inactive plantar (toe down)/dorsiflex (toe up)	▪ Focus on balls of feet ▪ Remove built-up heeled shoes ▪ Practise plantar/dorsiflex skip ▪ Ensure there is a slight forward body lean ▪ Keep head up; do not sink into the hips
Relaxation ▪ Relaxed ▪ Calm ▪ Comfortable	▪ Tense ▪ Too loose ▪ Distracted	▪ Imagine accelerating quickly with power and grace, but being calm and relaxed ▪ Breathing to be controlled

LATERAL STEPPING AND RUNNING

Correct	Incorrect	Solution
Foot action ▪ Work off balls of the feet	▪ On the heels ▪ Flat-footed	▪ Lean slightly forwards even when stepping sideways ▪ Provide constant feedback to keep off heels ▪ Keep hips tall and strong, this helps control power and prevent flat-footed weight transfer
▪ Feet shoulder-width apart	▪ Too wide ▪ Too close ▪ Crossed ▪ Pointing in	▪ Use marker spots to indicate best foot position for lateral stepping ▪ Practise stepping slowly at first, build up speed gradually ▪ Use marker spots to indicate best foot positions ▪ Use coloured tape, stick from tongue to end of shoes in straight line; working in front of mirror, focus on keeping the lines on the foot straight
▪ Drive off trailing foot	▪ Reach with leading foot ▪ Flat-footed ▪ Splayed out ▪ On heels ▪ Feet pointing in or splayed	▪ Place taped ball of paper under heel of each foot ▪ Use angled boards to step off
Hips ▪ Firm ▪ Controlled ▪ Square ▪ High	▪ Soft ▪ Twisted ▪ Angled ▪ Leaning too far forwards ▪ Bent at the waist ▪ Sunk	▪ Hold head tall ▪ Hold stomach in ▪ Focus on keeping hips square

LATERAL STEPPING AND RUNNING (continued)

Correct	Incorrect	Solution
Arms ■ Elbows at 90-degree angle ■ Fast and strong drive	■ Arm across the body ■ No arm drive at all ■ Arms too tight and restricted ■ Arms moving forwards but not driving backwards behind the hips	■ Constant positive feedback
Trunk ■ Strong and firm ■ Slight lean forwards	■ Too upright ■ Leaning too far forwards ■ Bent at the waist ■ Leaning back	■ Mirror drills ■ Head facing forward and still ■ Hold stomach in ■ Slight knee bend only

LATERAL TURNING – 90 DEGREES (PRE-TURN)

Correct	Incorrect	Solution
Feet ■ Shoulder-width apart	■ Together ■ Too wide ■ Crossed	■ Use chalk marks or marker spots to indicate best starting and finishing position
On the turn ■ Keep feet shoulder-width apart ■ Work on balls of feet	■ Come together ■ Cross ■ Too wide apart ■ On the heels ■ On the toes	■ Use chalk marks or marker spots to indicate best starting and finishing position ■ Practise single turn in front of mirror
Foot drive ■ Drive off trailing foot	■ Forward reach ■ Jump on the spot ■ Rock back on heels	■ Keep trunk firm ■ Get individuals to say the words, 'push' on the drive, 'off' on the turn, either in their heads or out loud ■ Practise lateral sidesteps slowly then build up speed ■ Maintain good arm drive

LIBRARY, UNIVERSITY OF CHESTER

TURNING LATERAL – 90 DEGREES (PRE–TURN)

Correct	Incorrect	Solution
Hips ■ High, slightly forwards ■ Hip before knee	■ Hip low and sunk ■ Angled not square ■ Trunk leaning too far forwards or too upright	■ Keep hips firm, tall and leaning forwards ■ Use arm drive with hips to assist turn ■ Keep hips square when turning ■ Practise turns slowly at first
Head ■ Keep up ■ Off the chest ■ Eyes looking forwards ■ Head and hip work simultaneously during turn	■ Floppy ■ Down ■ Angled ■ Back	■ Pick two distant objects, one in front of you, the other in the direction you are turning to. Initially focus on the object in front, on the turn refocus on the second object

180-DEGREE TURN

Correct	Incorrect	Solution
Initial Movement ■ Seamless ■ Movement smooth, no punctuations ■ Sequence is drop, step and go (1 – 2 – 3)	■ Jump up ■ Step back ■ Step forward ■ Twist and cross feet over	■ Practise drop step, the opening of the leg to point in the direction of the turn; the trailing foot then pushes off ■ Practise saying out loud 'drop, step and go' ■ Practise slowly at first, gradually developing speed ■ Practise facing a wall, so when you turn, the back step is prevented ■ Practise turn in front of mirror ■ Use video of turn
Feet ■ Shoulder-width apart	■ Together ■ Too wide ■ Crossed	■ Use chalk marks or marker spots to indicate best starting and finishing position
Arm drive ■ Elbows at 90-degree angle ■ Fast and strong drive	■ Arms across the body ■ No arm drive at all ■ Arms too tight and restricted ■ Arms moving forwards but not driving backwards behind the hips	■ Constant positive feedback
Head ■ Up ■ Eyes looking forwards	■ Down ■ Angled ■ Turned	■ Pick two distant objects, one in front of you, the other behind. Initially focus on the object in front, on the turn refocus on the second object (behind)
Hips ■ Hips, slightly forward and square ■ Hip before knee	■ Hip low and sunk ■ Angled not square ■ Trunk leaning too far forwards or too upright	■ Keep hips firm, tall and leaning forwards ■ Use arm drive with hips to assist turn ■ Hips kept square when turning ■ Practise turns slowly at first

JUMPING

Correct	Incorrect	Solution
Arm drive ■ Arms at 90 degrees, working together from behind the hips to above the head	■ No arm movement ■ Arms not working together ■ One arm used	■ Practise with a balloon; hold it in front, below the chest, with both hands, and then throw the balloon over the back of the head ■ Once balloon drill is perfected introduce the throwing of the balloon with a jump ■ Show the differences of jumping with arm drive and then without arm drive; attempt a jump with arms at the side then repeat with positive arm action
Pre-jump hips ■ Tall, slightly forwards	■ Bent ■ Sunk (most common)	■ Keep hips firm, tall and leaning forward ■ Keep hips square when jumping ■ Hold head up and stomach in
Take-off feet ■ Balls of the feet	■ Flat footed ■ On the heels ■ On the toes	■ Provide constant feedback to keep off heels ■ Keep hips tall and strong: this helps control power and prevent flat-footed weight transfer ■ Use a small, round stick or old book half an inch thick; place under both heels so that weight is forced onto the ball of the foot and practise jumping from this position
Landing ■ Balls of the feet ■ Weight equally balanced on both feet when possible	■ On the toes ■ On the heels ■ Unbalanced	■ Practise multiple bunny hops, landing on the balls of the feet, so that correct foot-to-ground contact is practised ■ Place taped ball of paper (size of a marble) under heel of each foot ■ Draw small circles or use small marker spots, between 2–3 inches in diameter and use these for landing markers for the balls of the feet
Trunk ■ Tall, hips slightly ` leaning forwards ■ Firm and relaxed	■ Sunk ■ Bent at the waist ■ Twisted ■ Uncontrolled	■ Breathe in and hold stomach firm, keeping head high
Hips ■ Firm ■ Tall ■ Slightly leaning forwards	■ Hip low and sunk ■ Angled not square ■ Trunk leaning too far forwards or too upright	■ Keep hips firm, tall and leaning forward ■ Use arm drive with hips to assist control ■ Keep hips square when landing ■ Practise landing by simply jumping off a step or small box ■ Imagine perfect body position

DECELERATION

Correct	Incorrect	Solution
Arms ■ Held at 90 degrees ■ Increase speed of drive on deceleration	■ Slow arm drive ■ No arm drive ■ Arms dropped by the sides	■ Provide feedback of 'drive arms' as soon as deceleration commences ■ Loop string or elastic bands around index finger and thumb and point of elbow to hold correct position of 90 degrees ■ Use light hand weights that are released on the deceleration phase
Feet ■ Shorten stride to smaller steps	■ Maintain long strides	■ Use coloured canes or marker dots or a short piece of outdoor Fast Foot Ladder on the deceleration phase
Head ■ Slightly raised above horizontal plane ■ Eyes up	■ Chin down on chest ■ Head turned to one side	■ Prior to deceleration phase pick object in the distance that is slightly higher than horizontal, requiring the head to be brought up ■ Teacher/coach to call 'head up' as deceleration phase begins
Hips ■ Lean back	■ Angled forward ■ Lopsided ■ Sunk or twisted	■ Focus on the head being brought up; this will change the angle of the hips

Trunk
■ Brought upright
	■ Remained tilted forwards
	■ Bent
		■ Get youngster to focus on:
		  1. Head up
		  2. Trunk up
		  3. Hips back
		Work on this combination during deceleration

Heel
■ Transfer weight to heel
■ Heel first
	■ On the toes
	■ Too much weight forwards on the balls of the feet
		■ Get athlete to focus on:
		  1. Head up
		  2. Trunk up
		  3. Hips back
		Work on this combination during deceleration. This will also impact on the spine and transfer to the heel coming down to the ground first for deceleration

DRILL ARM MECHANICS – ARM DRIVE

Aim
To perfect and practise correct arm technique for running.

Area/equipment
Indoor or outdoor area. Individual space to perform exercise.

Description
Youngsters stand with space around them so that they can perform the drill safely. Elbows are held at 90 degrees, hands relaxed; slowly the youngster brushes the inside of the wrist against the side of the body so that the elbow is driven back; the hand is then moved forward to the side of the face and returned to drive the elbow back again. Hips are kept square and head held up. Start very slowly and gradually build up speed.

Key teaching points
- Arms should not move across the body
- Forearms should not be chopped up and down as if hitting a drum
- Hands and shoulders should be relaxed
- Hips to be kept firm, not turned or twisted
- Head to be kept up on a horizontal plane
- Lean slightly forward onto the balls of the feet
- Keep core firm, do not sink into the hips.

Sets and reps
3 sets of 10 reps on each arm, 30 seconds recovery between each set.

Variation/progression
Youngster to hold foam ball in each hand, balls to be brushed against the side of the body (pocket area) and to the side of the cheek.

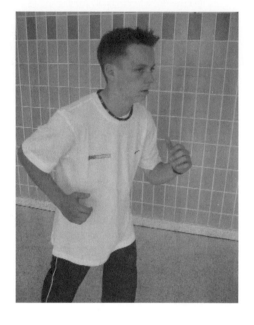

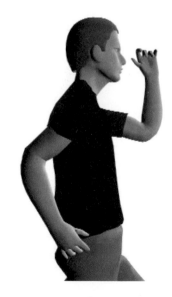

Figure 2.1 Arm mechanics – arm drive

DRILL ARM MECHANICS – PARTNER DRILLS

Aim
To perfect the correct arm technique for running.

Area/equipment
Youngster to work with a partner.

Description
Youngster stands with partner behind him or her. Partner holds the palms of his or her hands in line with the youngster's elbows, fingers pointing upwards. Youngster fires the arms as if sprinting, so that the elbows smack into partner's palms.

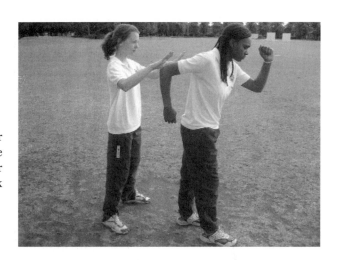

Key teaching points
- Arms should not move across the body
- Elbows should be at 90 degrees
- Hands and shoulders should be relaxed
- The insides of the wrists should brush against the pockets
- ROM – the hands should move from buttock cheeks to chest or head
- Encourage speed of movement to hear the smack.

Sets and reps
3 sets of 10 reps, with 30 seconds recovery between each set.

Variation/progression
Use beanbags or foam balls in each hand.

DRILL ARM MECHANICS – ARM DRIVE FOR JUMPING

Aim
To perfect correct arm technique for jumping.

Area/equipment
Indoor or outdoor area. Individual space to perform exercise.

Description
Youngsters stand with space around them so that they can perform the drill safely. Elbows are held at 90 degrees and hands are relaxed. Simultaneously both arms are slowly driven back so that they brush the side of the body with the side of the wrists.

Then at the same time they are brought forward to touch the side of the cheeks and then driven back slowly to the original position. Gradually increase the speed of the movement.

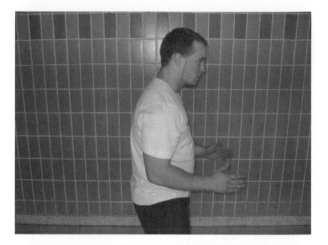

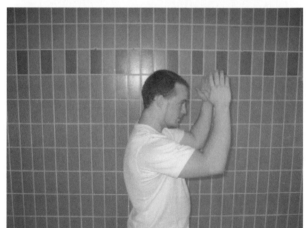

Key teaching points
■ Arms should not move across the body
■ Arms move together through an arc from hips to ears
■ Hands should be relaxed
■ Head to be held up
■ Use only a slight bend of the knees.

Sets and reps
3 sets of 10 reps, with 30 seconds recovery between each set.

Variation/progression
Use beanbags or foam balls in each hand.

DRILL | **ARM MECHANICS – BUTTOCK BOUNCE**

Aim
To develop explosive arm drive.

Area/equipment
Suitable ground surface.

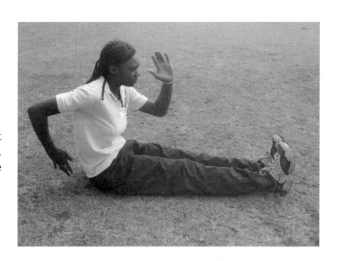

Description
Youngster sits on the floor with his/her legs straight out in front and fires his or her arms rapidly in short bursts. The power generated should be great enough to raise the buttocks off the floor in a bouncing manner.

Key teaching points
- Arms should not move across the body
- Elbows should be at 90 degrees
- Hands and shoulders should be relaxed
- The insides of the wrists should brush against the pockets
- ROM – the hands should move from buttock cheeks to chest or head
- Encourage speed of movement to hear the smack.

Sets and reps
2 sets of 4 reps; each rep is 6–8 explosive arm drives with 1 minute recovery between each set.

Variation/progression
Use beanbags or foam balls in each hand.

DRILL LEG MECHANICS – KNEE-LIFT DEVELOPMENT

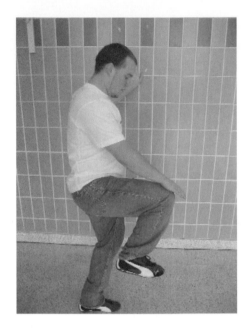

Aim
To develop and practise correct knee-lift technique for running.

Area/equipment
Indoor or outdoor area. Fence, wall or partner to lean against.

Description
Youngster leans against wall with one arm, the other arm is angled down so that the palm (facing down) is just below the waist out in front of the body. Knee is brought up to the palm of hand and then down, ensuring that the ball of the foot and not the heel hits the ground. This is repeated on both sides of the body.

Key teaching points
- Start slowly. gradually increase speed
- Knee to be brought up to the horizontal
- Ball of the foot, not any other part of the foot, to hit the ground
- Get youngster to look ahead
- Body should lean slightly
- No sinking or twisting of the hips.

Sets and reps
2 sets of 10 reps on each leg, 30 seconds recovery between each set.

Variations/progressions
- Hold arm out above the waist, which will vary the height of the knee-lift
- Use mats, carpet, foam so that the foot strikes the material, providing a different feedback to the youngster.

DRILL | RUNNING FORM – DEAD-LEG RUN

Aim
To develop a quick knee-lift and the positive foot placement required for effective sprinting.

Area/equipment
Indoor or outdoor area. Using hurdles, marker dots or sticks, place approximately 8 obstacles in a straight line at 2–foot intervals. Place a marker dot 1 yard from each end of the line to mark a start and finish.

Description
Youngster must keep the outside leg straight in a locked position. The inside leg moves over the obstacles in a cycling motion while the outside leg swings along just above the ground.

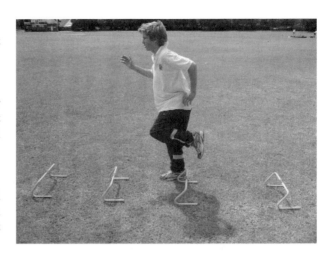

Key teaching points
- Bring the knee of the inside leg up to just below 90 degrees
- Point the toe upwards
- Bring the inside leg back down quickly between the hurdles
- Increase the speed when the technique has been mastered
- Maintain correct arm mechanics
- Maintain an upright posture and a strong core
- Keep the hips square and stand tall.

Sets and reps
1 set of 6 reps, 3 leading with the left leg and 3 with the right.

Variation/progression
Place several different-coloured markers 2 yards from the last hurdle at different angles. As the youngster leaves the last hurdle the teacher/coach nominates a marker for the youngster to accelerate to.

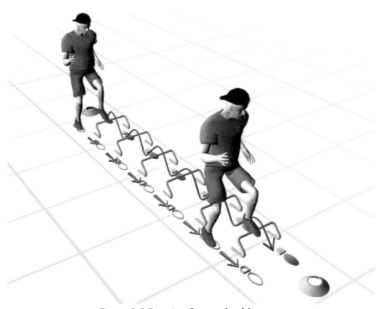

Figure 2.2 Running form – dead-leg run

DRILL   *RUNNING FORM – PRE-TURN*

Aim

To educate and prepare the hips, legs and feet for effective and quick turning without fully committing the whole body.

Area/equipment

Indoor or outdoor area. Using hurdles, marker dots or sticks, place about 8 obstacles in a straight line at 2-foot intervals. Place a marker dot 1 yard from each end of the line to mark a start and finish.

Description

Youngster moves sideways along the line of obstacles, just in front of them, i.e. not travelling over them. The back leg (following leg) is brought over the hurdle to a position slightly in front of the body so that the heel is in line with the toe of the leading foot. As the back foot is planted, the leading foot moves away. Repeat the drill leading with the opposite leg.

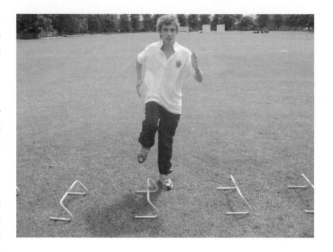

Key teaching points

■ Stand tall and do not sink into the hips
■ Do not allow the feet to cross over
■ Keep the feet shoulder-width apart as much as possible
■ The knee-lift should be no greater than 45 degrees
■ Maintain correct arm mechanics
■ Maintain an upright posture
■ Keep the hips and shoulders square
■ Work both the left and right sides.

Sets and reps

1 set of 6 reps, 3 with the left shoulder and 3 with the right.

Variations/progressions

■ Place several different-coloured markers 2 yards from the last hurdle at different angles. As the youngster leaves the last hurdle the teacher/coach nominates a marker for the youngster to accelerate to
■ Work two youngsters opposite one another and place a ball approximately 5 yards from the last hurdle. As the youngsters leave the last hurdle each races to get to the ball before the other.

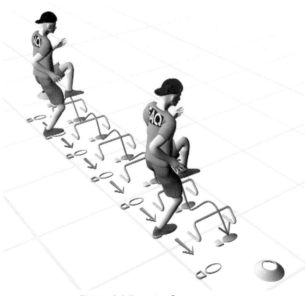

Figure 2.3 Running form – pre-turn

DRILL   *RUNNING FORM – LEADING-LEG RUN*

Aim
To develop quick, efficient steps and running techniques.

Area/equipment
Indoor or outdoor area. Using hurdles, marker dots or sticks, place approximately 8 obstacles in a straight line at 2-foot intervals. Place a marker dot 1 yard from each end of the line to mark a start and finish.

Description
Youngster runs down the line of obstacles, crossing over each one with the same lead leg. The aim is to just clear the obstacles. Repeat the drill using the opposite leg as the lead.

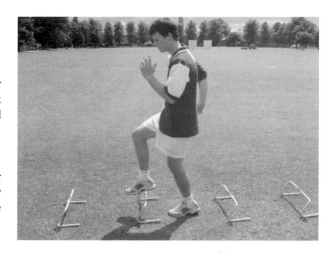

Key teaching points
- The knee-lift should be no more than 45 degrees
- Use short, sharp steps
- Maintain strong arm mechanics
- Maintain an upright posture
- Stand tall and do not sink into the hips

Sets and reps
1 set of 4 reps, 2 leading with the left leg and 2 with the right.

Variations/progressions
- A good exercise for changing direction after running in a straight line is to place 3 marker dots at the end of the obstacles at different angles 2–3 metres away; on leaving the last obstacle, the youngster sprints out to the marker dot nominated by the teacher/coach
- Vary the distance between the hurdles to achieve different stride lengths

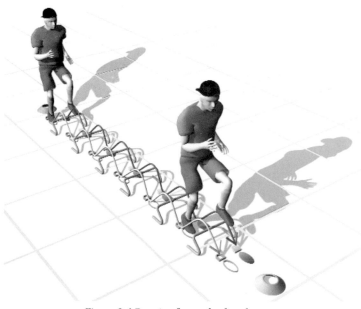

Figure 2.4 Running form – leading-leg run

| **DRILL** | *RUNNING FORM – QUICK SIDESTEP DEVELOPMENT*

Aim
To develop correct, precise and controlled lateral stepping movements.

Area/equipment
Indoor or outdoor area. Place 3 hurdles side by side about 18 inches apart.

Description
Youngster stands on the outside of either hurdle 1 or hurdle 3 so that he or she will step over the middle of each hurdle. The youngster performs lateral mechanics movement while clearing each hurdle; on clearing hurdle 3 he or she repeats the drill in the opposite direction.

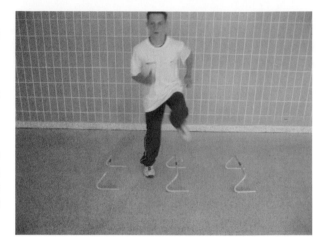

Key teaching points
- Maintain correct lateral running form/mechanics
- Maintain correct arm mechanics
- Do not sink into the hips
- Keep the head up
- Do not lean too far forwards
- Use small steps and work off the balls of the feet
- Do not use an excessively high knee-lift.

Sets and reps
2 sets of 10 reps, 5 to the left and 5 to the right with 1 minute recovery between sets.

Variations/progressions
- Work with a teacher/coach, who should randomly direct the youngster over the marker dots
- Add 2 Macro V Hurdles to add lift variation.

DRILL | *RUNNING FORM – SIDESTEP DEVELOPMENT*

Aim
To develop efficient and economical lateral sidesteps.

Area/equipment
Indoor or outdoor area. Place 8 Micro V Hurdles side on, 1 yard apart and staggered laterally. Position a finish marker dot in the same pattern as the hurdles.

Description
Youngster works inside the channel created by the hurdles, stepping over each hurdle with one foot as he or she moves laterally down and across the channel, and on reaching the end of the channel, walks back to the start and repeats the drill.

Key teaching points
- Bring the knee up 45 degrees over the hurdle
- Do not overstride across the hurdle
- Maintain correct arm mechanics / strong arm drive
- Keep the hips square
- Do not sink into the hips.

Sets and reps
2 sets of 3 reps with a walk-back recovery between reps and 2 minutes between sets.

Variation/progression
Perform the drill backwards.

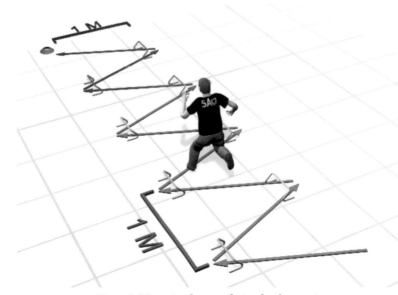

Figure 2.5 Running form – sidestep development

DRILL   RUNNING FORM – LATERAL STEP

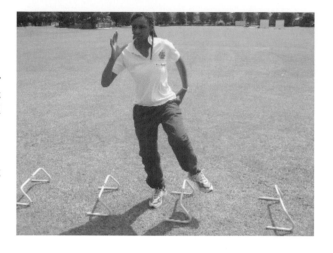

Aim
To develop efficient and economical lateral steps.

Area/equipment
Indoor or outdoor area. Using hurdles, marker dots or sticks, place approximately 8 obstacles in a straight line at 2-foot intervals. Place a marker dot 1 yard from each end of the line to mark a start and finish.

Description
Youngster steps over each obstacle while moving sideways.

Key teaching points
- Bring the knee up to just below 45 degrees
- Do not skip sideways – step!
- Push off from the back foot
- Do not pull with the lead foot
- Maintain correct arm mechanics
- Maintain an upright posture
- Keep the hips square
- Do not sink into the hips.

Sets and reps
1 set of 6 reps, 3 leading with left shoulder and 3 with the right.

Variation/progression
Place several different-coloured markers 2 yards from the last hurdle at different angles. As the youngster leaves the last hurdle the teacher/coach nominates a marker for him or her to accelerate to.

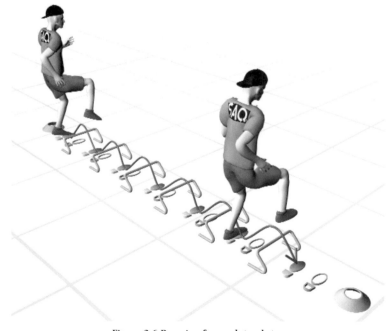

Figure 2.6 Running form – lateral step

| DRILL | *RUNNING FORM – 1-2-3 LIFT* |

Aim
To develop an efficient leg cycle, rhythm, power and foot placement.

Area/equipment
Indoor or outdoor area 20–25 yards long, marker dots.

Description
Youngster moves in a straight line and after every third step the leg is brought up in an explosive action to 90 degrees. Continue the drill over the length prescribed working the same leg and then repeat the drill leading with the other leg. Marker dots can be placed to mark the spot where the leg is brought up explosively.

Key teaching points
- Keep the hips square
- Work off the balls of the feet
- Try to develop and maintain a rhythm
- Keep eyes and head up and look ahead
- Maintain correct arm mechanics
- Maintain an upright posture.

Sets and reps
1 set of 4 reps, 2 leading with the left leg and 2 with the right.

Variations/progressions
- Alternate the lead leg during a repetition
- Vary the lift sequence, e.g. 1-2-3-4-lift, etc.

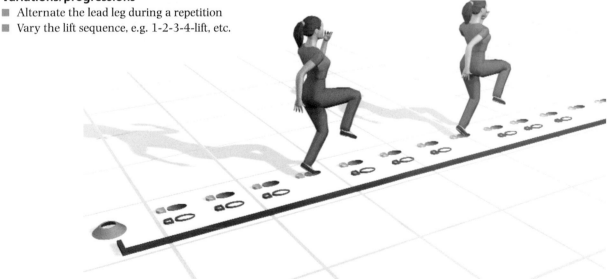

Figure 2.7 Running form – 1-2-3 lift

DRILL JUMPING – SINGLE JUMPS

Aim
To develop jumping techniques, power, speed and control.

Area/equipment
Indoor or outdoor area. Ensure the surface is clear of any obstacles.
Use 7-or-12 inch hurdles.

Description
Youngster jumps over a single hurdle and on landing walks back to the
start point to repeat the drill.

Key teaching points
■ Maintain good arm mechanics
■ Do not sink into the hips at the take-off and landing phases
■ Land on the balls of the feet
■ Do not fall back on the heels.

Sets and reps
2 sets of 4 reps with 1 minute recovery between each set.

Variations/progression
Introduce stability work, youngster to hold position on landing.

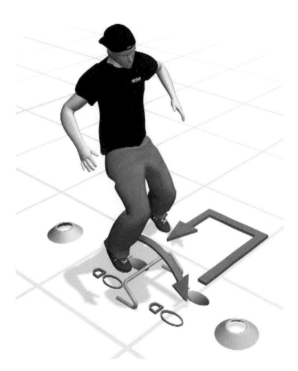

Figure 2.8 Jumping – single jumps

DRILL   *JUMPING – SINGLE JUMPS OVER AND BACK*

Aim
To develop jumping techniques, power, speed and control.

Area/equipment
Indoor or outdoor area. Ensure the surface is clear of any obstacles.
Marker dots.

Description
Youngster jumps over a single hurdle and on landing turns and jumps
back over the hurdle to repeat the drill.

Key teaching points
- Maintain good arm mechanics
- Do not sink into the hips at the take-off and landing phases
- Land on the balls of the feet
- Do not fall back on the heels.

Sets and reps
2 sets of 4 reps with 1 minute recovery between each set.

Variation/progression
Introduce stability work, youngster to hold position
on landing.

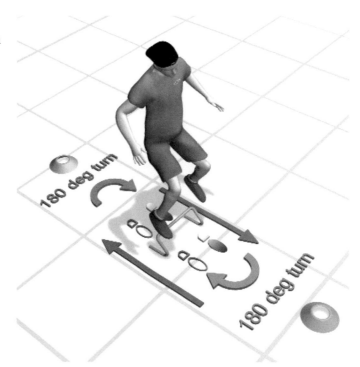

Figure 2.9 Jumping – single jumps over and back

DRILL   *JUMPING – SINGLE JUMP WITH 180-DEGREE TWIST*

Aim
To develop jumping techniques, power, speed and control.

Area/equipment
Indoor or outdoor area. Ensure the surface is clear of any obstacles.
Use 4, 7 or 12 inch hurdles.

Description
Youngster jumps and twists 180 degrees over a single hurdle and on
landing walks back to the start point to repeat the drill.

Key teaching points
- Maintain good arm mechanics
- Do not sink into the hips at the take-off and landing phases
- Land on the balls of the feet
- Do not fall back on the heels.

Sets and reps
2 sets of 4 reps with 1 minute recovery between each set.

Variation/progression
Introduce stability work, youngsters hold position on landing.

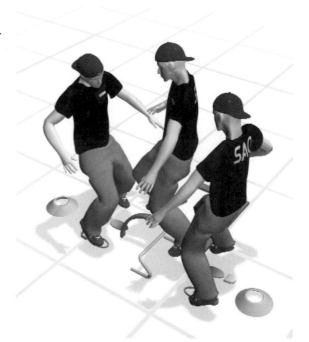

Figure 2.10 Jumping – single jump with 180-degree twist

DRILL   *JUMPING – LATERAL SINGLE JUMPS*

Aim
To develop jumping techniques, power, speed and control.

Area/equipment
Indoor or outdoor area. Ensure the surface is clear of any obstacles.
Use 4, 7 or 12 inch hurdles.

Description
Youngster jumps laterally over a single hurdle and on landing walks
back to the start point to repeat the drill.

Key teaching points
- Maintain good arm mechanics
- Do not sink into the hips at the take-off and landing phases
- Land on the balls of the feet
- Do not fall back on the heels.

Sets and reps
2 sets of 4 reps with 1 minute recovery between each set.

Variations/progressions
- Introduce stability work, youngster holds position on
  landing.
- Youngster to jump laterally over and back.

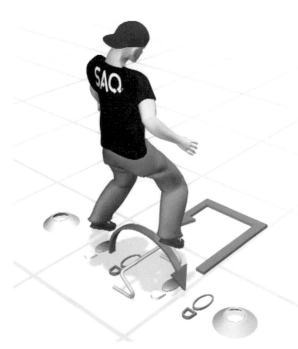

Figure 2.11 Jumping – lateral single jumps

FORWARD JUMP – MULTIPLE JUMPS

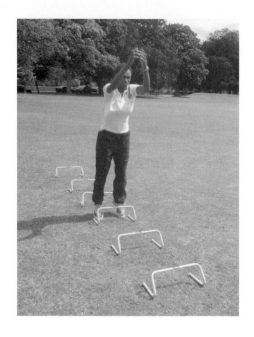

Aim
To develop maximum control while taking off and landing. To develop controlled directional power.

Area/equipment
Indoor or outdoor area. Place 6–8 hurdles of 4, 7 or 12 inches in height at 2-foot intervals in a straight line.

Description
Youngster jumps forward over each hurdle in quick succession until all hurdles have been cleared, then walks back to the start and repeats the drill.

Key teaching points
- Use quick, rhythmic arm mechanics
- Do not sink into the hips at the take-off and landing phases
- Land and take off from the balls of the feet
- Stand tall and look straight ahead
- Maintain control
- Gradually build up the speed.

Sets and reps
2 sets of 6 reps with 1 minute recovery between each set.

Variation/progression
Introduce stability, youngster to hold position after each jump.

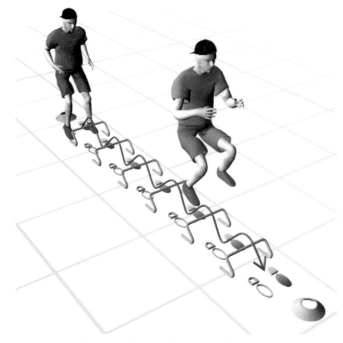

Figure 2.12 Forward jump – multiple jumps

DRILL   *LATERAL JUMP – MULTIPLE JUMPS*

Aim
To develop maximum control while taking off and landing. To develop controlled directional power.

Area/equipment
Indoor or outdoor area. Place 6–8 hurdles of 4, 7 or 12 inches at 2 foot intervals in a straight line.

Description
Youngster jumps laterally over each hurdle in quick succession until all hurdles have been cleared, then walks back to the start and repeats the drill.

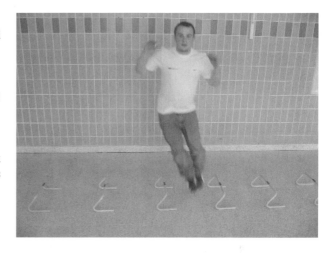

Key teaching points
- Use quick, rhythmic arm mechanics
- Do not sink into the hips at the take-off and landing phases
- Land and take off from the balls of the feet
- Stand tall and look straight ahead
- Maintain control
- Gradually build up the speed.

Sets and reps
2 sets of 6 reps with 1 minute recovery between each set.

Variation/progression
Introduce stability, youngster to hold position on landing.

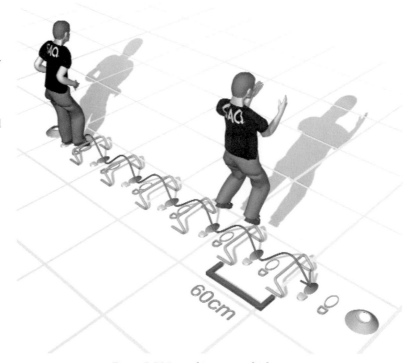

Figure 2.13 Lateral jump – multiple jumps

DRILL — HOP JUMPS – MULTIPLE HOPS

Aim
To develop maximum control while taking off and landing. To develop controlled directional power.

Area/equipment
Indoor or outdoor area. Place 6–8 hurdles of 4, 7 or 12 inches in height at 2-foot intervals in a straight line.

Description
Youngster hops over each hurdle in quick succession until all hurdles have been cleared, then walks back to the start and repeats the drill.

Key teaching points
- Use quick, rhythmic arm mechanics
- Do not sink into the hips at the take-off and landing phases
- Land and take off from the balls of the feet
- Stand tall and look straight ahead
- Maintain control
- Gradually build up the speed.

Sets and reps
2 sets of 6 reps with 1 minute recovery between each set.

Variations/progressions
- Alternate landing and take-off foot
- Introduce stability, hold position on landing then repeat.

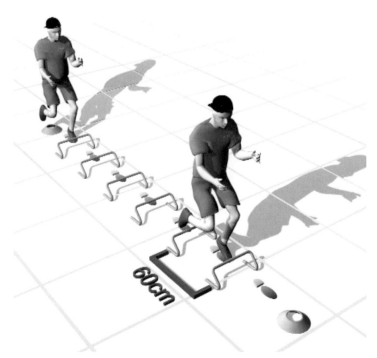

Figure 2.14 Hop jumps – multiple hops

DRILL | *180-DEGREE TWIST JUMPS – MULTIPLE JUMPS*

Aim

To develop maximum control while taking off and landing. To develop controlled directional power.

Area/equipment

Indoor or outdoor area. Place 6–8 hurdles of 4, 7 or 12 inches at 2-foot intervals in a straight line.

Description

Youngster jumps and twists 180 degrees over each hurdle in quick succession until all hurdles have been cleared, then walks back to the start and repeats the drill.

Key teaching points

- Use quick, rhythmic arm mechanics
- Do not sink into the hips at the take-off and landing phases
- Land and take off from the balls of the feet
- Stand tall and look straight ahead
- Maintain control
- Gradually build up the speed.

Sets and reps

2 sets of 6 reps with 1 minute recovery between each set.

Variations/progressions

- Introduce stability, hold position on landing
- Introduce alternate twisting over each hurdle.

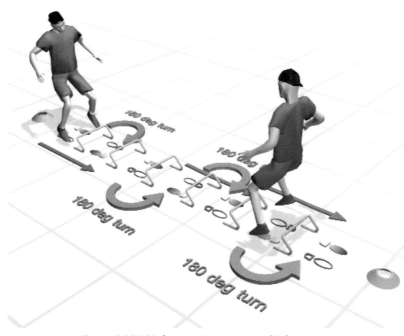

Figure 2.15 180-degree twist jumps – multiple jumps

DRILL

RUNNING FORM –
STRIDE FREQUENCY AND STRIDE LENGTH

Aim

To practise the transfer from the acceleration phase to an increase in stride frequency and length required when running – to develop an efficient leg cycle, rhythm, power and foot placement.

Area/equipment

Indoor or outdoor area, 20–30 yards long. Place 12 coloured 4-foot sticks or canes flat on the ground at 5–6-foot intervals (the intervals will be determined by the size and age of the group).

Description

Starting 10 yards away from the first stick the youngster accelerates towards the sticks and aims to land just past each one. After the last stick the youngster gradually decelerates. He or she returns to the start and repeats the drill.

Key teaching points

- Do not overstride
- Work off the balls of the feet
- Try to develop and maintain a rhythm
- Keep eyes and head up as if looking over a fence
- Maintain correct mechanics
- Maintain an upright posture
- Stay focused
- Alter distances between strides for different ages and heights.

Sets and reps

1 set of 3 reps.

Variations/progressions

- Set up the stride frequency sticks as shown in figure 2.16. The sticks now control the acceleration and deceleration phases
- Add change of direction during the deceleration phase
- After deceleration add stability skill by getting the youngsters to stand still for 3–4 seconds on the balls of the feet with their hands out in a defensive type position.

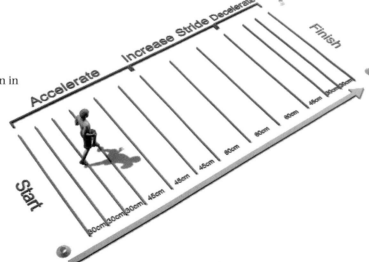

Figure 2.16 Running form – stride frequency and stride length

DRILL RUNNING FORM – HURDLE MIRROR DRILLS

Aim
To improve random agility; to challenge the youngster's ability to mirror another youngster's movements.

Area/equipment
Indoor or outdoor area. Mark out a grid with 2 lines of 8 hurdles or marker dots with 2 feet between each hurdle and 2 yards between each line of hurdles.

Description
Youngsters face each other while performing mechanics drills up and down the lines of hurdles. One youngster initiates the movements while the partner attempts to mirror them. Youngsters can perform both lateral and linear mirror drills.

Key teaching points
- Stay focused on partner
- The youngster mirroring should try to anticipate the lead youngster's movements
- Maintain correct arm mechanics.

Sets and reps
Each youngster performs 3 sets of 30-second work periods. Ensure 30 seconds recovery between each work period.

Variations/progressions
- First-to-the-marker-dot – as above, except a ball is placed between the 2 lines of hurdles. The proactive partner commences the drill as normal then accelerates to touch the dot, while the reactive youngster attempts to beat the proactive youngster to the dot.
- Lateral drills performed as above – youngsters work in pairs with only 2 hurdles each: effective for improving short-stepping, lateral skills.

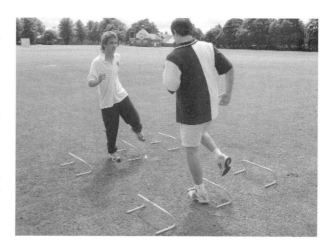

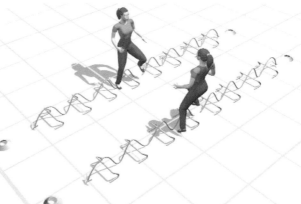

Figure 2.17(a) Hurdle mirror drills

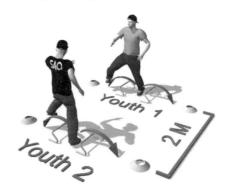

Figure 2.17(b) Hurdle mirror drills – two hurdles each

DRILL   *RUNNING FORM – COMPLEX MECHANICS*

Aim
To prevent youngsters resorting to bad habits particularly when under pressure; to challenge youngsters by placing them in game-like pressure situations; to maintain good running form even in the most difficult and demanding of situations.

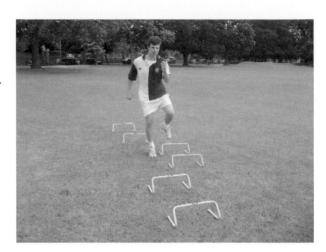

Area/equipment
Indoor or outdoor area. Place 4 hurdles in a straight line with 2 feet between each hurdle. The next 4 hurdles are set slightly to one side, and the final 4 hurdles are placed back in line with the original 4.

Description
Youngsters performs a dead-leg run over the hurdles with the dead leg changing over the 4 centre hurdles. Return to the start by performing the drill over the hurdles in the opposite direction.

Key teaching points
- Maintain correct arm mechanics
- Work off the balls of the feet
- Try to develop and maintain a rhythm
- Keep eyes and head up and look ahead
- Maintain an upright posture
- Keep the hips square.

Sets and reps
4 sets of 4 reps.

Variations/progressions
- Perform the drill laterally, moving both forwards and backwards to cross the centre 4 hurdles
- Place hurdles in a cross formation and perform drills up to the centre and then sideways, left or right, up or across
- Introduce youngster from other sides/groups.

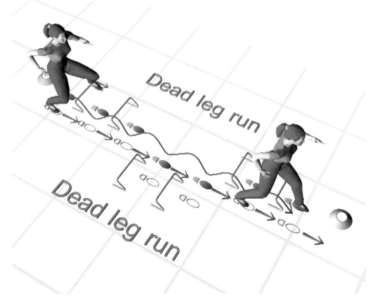

Figure 2.18 Running form `– complex mechanics

DRILL — *RUNNING FORM – CURVED ANGLE RUNS*

Aim
To develop controlled, explosive fast feet while running on a curved angle.

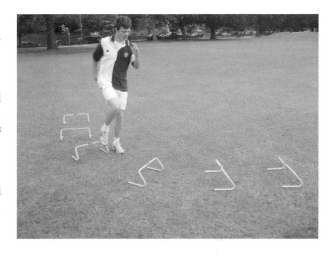

Area/equipment
Indoor or outdoor area. Place 10 hurdles in a curved formation, 2 feet apart. Place a marker dot at each end, approximately 2 yards from the first and last hurdles respectively.

Description
Youngster performs running drill as already described (Dead-Leg Run, Lateral Stepping or Leading Leg Run), with same leg leading over each hurdle.

Key teaching points
- Work both left and right sides
- The knee-lift should be no more than 45 degrees
- Use short, sharp steps
- Maintain powerful arm mechanics
- Maintain an upright posture
- Look ahead at all times.

Sets and reps
Each youngster performs 1 set of 4 reps. Leave 30 seconds recovery between each work rep.

Variations/progressions
- Introduce a foam ball
- Introduce stability, hold position momentarily after each step
- Introduce tighter curves
- Use immediately after straight run hurdle work.

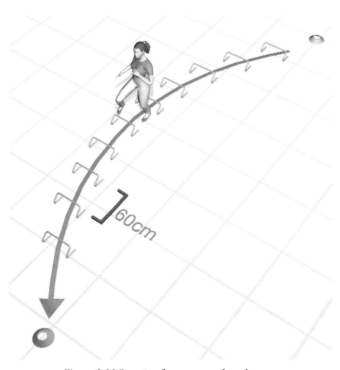

Figure 2.19 Running form – curved angle runs

RUNNING FORM –
THE SQUARE COMPLEX MECHANICS

Aim

To bring together running form drills into different combinations so that youngsters become more comfortable at changing movement patterns when required.

Area/equipment

Indoor or outdoor area. Place 4 lines of hurdles or marker dots in a square 2 feet apart.

Description

Youngster performs a different mechanics drill down each line of hurdles until the square is completed.

Key teaching points

- Maintain correct arm mechanics
- Work off the balls of the feet
- Try to develop and maintain a rhythm
- Keep eyes and head up and look ahead
- Maintain an upright posture
- Keep the hips square.

Sets and reps

2 sets of 4 reps.

Variation/progression

Vary the combination of sets of drills down each of the hurdles.

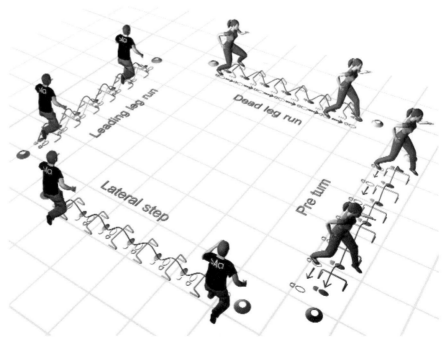

Figure 2.20 Running form – the square complex mechanics

CHAPTER 3 INNERVATION

INCREASING THE SPEED OF MOVEMENT

Innervation is the transition stage from warm-up and mechanics to periods of higher intensity of work that activate the neural pathways, or in more simple terms, cause the nerves to fire the muscle as quickly as possible. Faster moving hands, feet and body control enables youngsters to perform co-ordinated movements of speed and agility such as sidesteps, short explosive sprints, fast hands to catch and the quickness of turn and chase. The key in this section is to quicken the movements without compromising the quality of movement techniques. It is important to perfect the movement slowly then increase the intensity and quickness.

Health and safety

- Check spacing of ladders, i.e. create plenty of space at either end and between them

- Fatigue will lead to poor technique and slow feet

- Improved foot placement helps prevent foot and ankle injuries

- Never secure the ladders to the surface

- START SLOW before getting FAST

Developing and progressing ladder drills

- Vary direction of movement

- Alternate leading foot

- One foot moves quickly while the other is used for support

- Vary size of movements: use small ones inside the ladder, larger ones outside

- Add twists and turns

- Vary height of movements, both in stepping and jumping

- Change direction in and out of the ladder

- Use marker dots in the squares in the ladder to indicate change of movement or action

- Introduce stops and starts: this will help develop stability

- Incorporate ball skills (manipulation) out of the ladder, progress to ball skills in the ladder

- Youngsters to carry rackets or bats so that striking drills can be introduced in and out of the ladder.

DRILL FAST FOOT LADDER – SINGLE WALK

Aim
To develop awareness, confidence and familiarity with technique and equipment.

Area/equipment
Use an indoor or outdoor area. Use a Fast Foot Ladder – ensure that this is the correct ladder for the type of surface being used.

Description
Youngster covers the length of the ladder by placing a foot in each ladder space at a walking pace. Return to the start by walking back beside the ladder.

Key teaching points
■ Maintain correct form/mechanics
■ Ensure arms are at 90 degrees and are driven forwards and backwards at the right angle
■ Maintain an upright posture
■ Keep off the toes, encourage walking on the balls of the feet
■ Stress that quality not quantity is important.

Sets and reps
2 sets of 3 reps with 30 seconds recovery between each set.

Variation/progression
Single lateral walk.

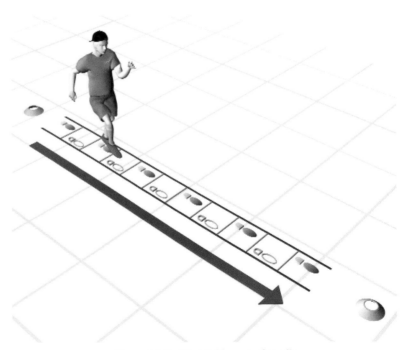

Figure 3.1 Fast foot ladder – single walk

DRILL — FAST FOOT LADDER – SINGLE RUN

Aim
To develop linear fast feet with control, precision and power.

Area/equipment
Use an indoor or outdoor area. Use a Fast Foot Ladder – ensure that this is the correct ladder for the type of surface being used.

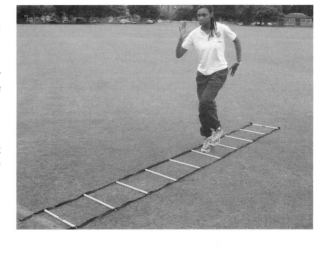

Description
Youngster covers the length of the ladder by placing a foot in each ladder space (see fig 3.2). Return to the start by jogging back beside the ladder.

Key teaching points
- Maintain correct running form/mechanics
- Start slowly and gradually increase the speed
- Maintain an upright posture
- Stress that quality not quantity is important.

Sets and reps
2 sets of 3 reps with 1 minute recovery between each set.

Variations/progressions
- Youngster to throw beanbag into one of the ladder squares, run and pick it up and continue running down the ladder
- Place a marker dot halfway down the ladder; when the youngster reaches the dot she or he stops, counts to three and starts again.
- Stability drill: place marker dot halfway down the ladder: when the youngster reaches the dot she or he stands on one foot and holds the position, counts to five and starts again.

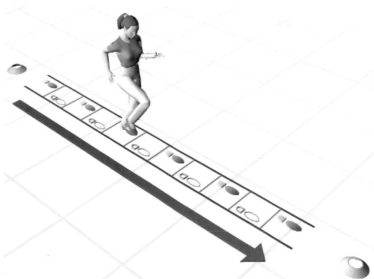

Figure 3.2 Fast foot ladder – single run

DRILL · FAST FOOT LADDER – SINGLE LATERAL STEPS

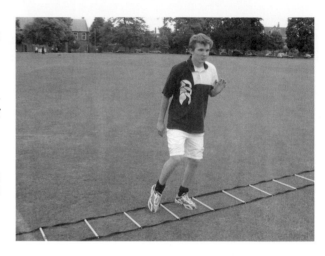

Aim
To develop lateral fast feet with control, precision and power.

Area/equipment
Use an indoor or outdoor area. Use a Fast Foot Ladder – ensure that this is the correct ladder for the type of surface being used.

Description
Youngster covers the length of the ladder moving sideways by placing a foot in each ladder space and returns to the start by jogging back beside the ladder.

Key teaching points
- Maintain correct running form/mechanics
- Start slowly and gradually increase the speed
- Maintain an upright posture
- Stress that quality not quantity is important
- Push off from the back foot.

Sets and reps
2 sets of 3 reps with 1 minute recovery between each set.

Variations/progressions
- Place a marker dot outside one of the ladder squares; when the youngster reaches the square directly opposite the marker dot, he or she steps out then steps back into the ladder, and continues the movement down the ladder
- Manipulation skills: on completing the ladder drill, a ball is provided so that youngsters can bounce the ball on the way back to the starting point.

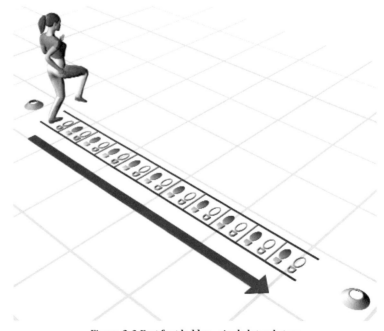

Figure 3.3 Fast foot ladder – single lateral steps

DRILL   *FAST FOOT LADDER – UP AND BACK*

Aim
To develop lateral stepping movement.

Area/equipment
Use indoor or outdoor area. Use a Fast Foot Ladder – ensure that this is the correct ladder for the type of surface being used.

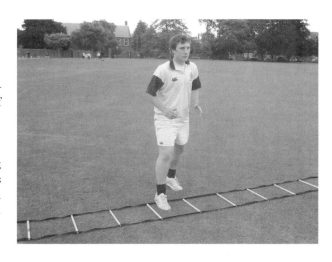

Description
Youngster covers the length of the ladder by moving laterally and, alternating forwards and backwards, steps in and out of the squares for the length of the ladder; then jogs back to the start and repeats with the other shoulder.

Key teaching points
- Maintain correct jumping/hopping form/mechanics
- Start slowly and gradually increase the speed
- Stress that quality not quantity is important
- Keep off the heels
- Do not let youngster sink into the hips.

Sets and reps
2 sets of 3 reps with 1 minute recovery between each set.

Variations/progressions
- Place a marker dot in one of the squares; this signals to the youngster to change legs
- Place marker dot halfway down the ladder; on landing on the dot the position is held for 5 seconds, helping to develop the youngster's stability.

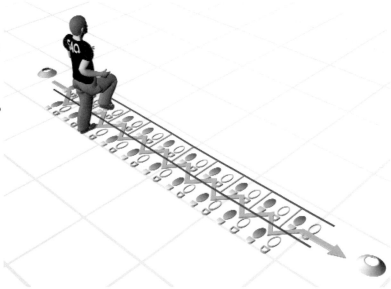

Figure 3.4 Fast foot ladder – up and back

DRILL   FAST FOOT LADDER – LATERAL STEP IN AND OUT

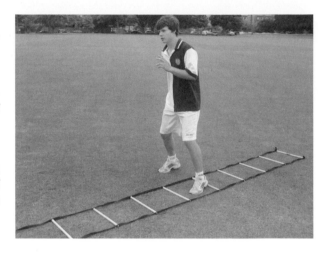

Aim
To develop laterally in-and-out fast feet with control, precision and power.

Area/equipment
Use an indoor or outdoor area. Use a Fast Foot Ladder – ensure that this is the correct ladder for the type of surface being used.

Description
Youngster to cover the length of the ladder by running down the side of the ladder and stepping in and out of each ladder space with the leg nearest the ladder. This is repeated on the other side.

Key teaching points
■ Maintain correct running form mechanics
■ Start slowly and gradually increase the speed
■ Maintain an upright posture
■ Keep head up and focus on an object on horizon.

Sets and reps
2 sets of 4 reps with 1 minute recovery between each set.

Variations/progressions
■ Introduce stepping into every second ladder space
■ Randomly place marker spot in ladder space for youngster to step in and out on.

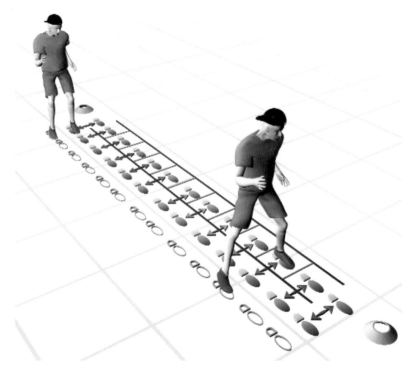

Figure 3.5 Fast foot ladder – lateral step in and out

DRILL FAST FOOT LADDER – SMALL DEAD-LEG RUN

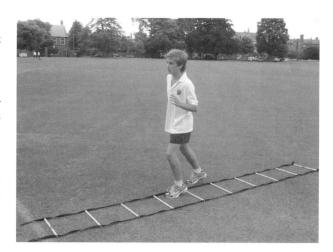

Aim
To develop quick, short knee-lift and positive foot placement for running.

Area/equipment
Use an indoor or outdoor area. Use a Fast Foot Ladder – ensure that the correct ladder for the type of surface is being used.

Description
Youngster works down the side of the ladder, keeping the outside leg straight in a locked position. The inside leg moves over the ladder rungs in a short fast cycle motion, while the outside leg swings along just above the ground.

Key teaching points
- Maintain correct arm mechanics
- Maintain an upright posture and strong core
- Keep the hips square and stand tall
- Only increase the speed when technique has been mastered
- Listen for too much sound from foot placement; this means youngster is hitting the floor with flat foot.

Sets and reps
2 sets of 4 reps with a 1 minute recovery between each set.

Variations/progressions
- Integrate step in, step out and Dead Leg Run
- Randomly place Macro V Hurdle in ladder square for higher knee-lift.

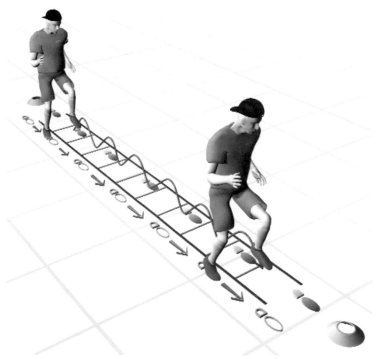

Figure 3.6 Fast foot ladder – small dead-leg run

DRILL   FAST FOOT LADDER – ICKY SHUFFLE

Aim
To develop controlled, balanced lateral movement.

Area/equipment
Use indoor or outdoor area. Use a Fast Foot Ladder – ensure that this is the correct ladder for the type of surface being used.

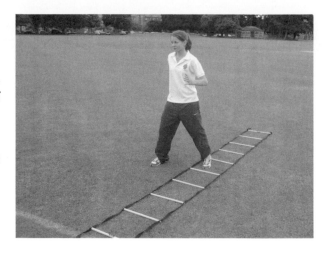

Description
Youngster covers the length of the ladder performing lateral footwork drill as shown in fig. 3.7.

Key teaching points
- Maintain correct lateral form/mechanics
- Start slowly and gradually increase the speed
- Stress that quality not quantity is important
- Keep off the heels
- Do not let youngster sink into hips
- Do not skip with both feet in the air.

Sets and reps
2 sets of 3 reps with 1 minute recovery between each set.

Variation/progression
Place a marker dot directly outside one of the ladder squares; when the youngster's outside foot steps on the marker dot the position is held for 3 seconds. This will help develop stability.

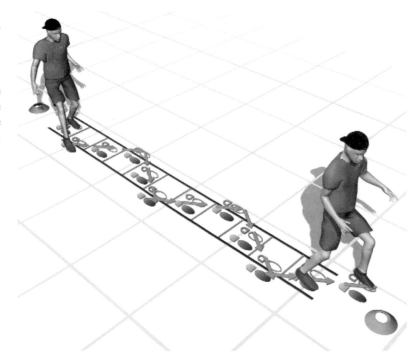

Figure 3.7 Fast foot ladder – icky shuffle

DRILL *FAST FOOT LADDER – DOUBLE RUN*

Aim
To develop very fast linear feet with control, precision and power.

Area/equipment
Indoor or outdoor area. Use a Fast Foot Ladder – ensure that this is the correct ladder for the type of surface being used.

Description
Youngster covers the length of the ladder by placing both feet in each ladder space (see fig 3.1). Return to the start by jogging back beside the ladder.

Key teaching points
■ Maintain correct running form/mechanics
■ Start slowly and gradually increase the speed
■ Maintain an upright posture
■ Stress that quality not quantity is important.

Sets and reps
2 sets of 3 reps with 1 minute recovery between each set.

Variations/progressions
■ Perform drill laterally; youngster to put both feet in each ladder space while moving sideways
■ Youngster to throw beanbag into one of the ladder squares, run and pick it up and continue running down the ladder
■ Place a marker dot halfway down the ladder; when the youngster reaches the dot she or he stops, counts to three and starts again
■ Stability drill: place marker dot halfway down the ladder; when the youngster reaches the dot she or he stands on one foot and holds the position for a count of five and starts again.

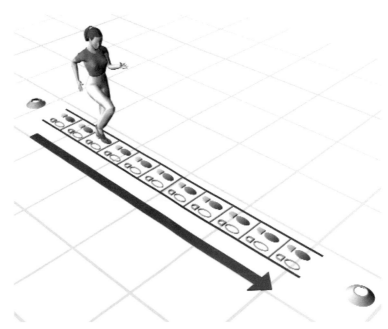

Figure 3.8 Fast foot ladder – double run

DRILL FAST FOOT LADDER – HOPSCOTCH

Aim

To develop combined jumping techniques, balance and co-ordination.

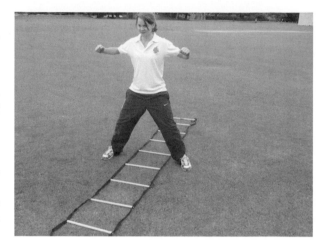

Area/equipment

Use an indoor or outdoor area. Use a Fast Foot Ladder – ensure that this is the correct ladder for the type of surface being used.

Description

Youngster covers the length of the ladder by jumping into one square with both feet together then into next square with feet on either side of it, repeating this along the ladder, then returns to the start by jogging back beside the ladder.

Key teaching points

- Maintain correct jumping form/mechanics
- Start slowly and gradually increase the speed
- Maintain an upright posture
- Stress that quality not quantity is important
- Keep off the heels.

Sets and reps

2 sets of 3 reps with 1 minute recovery between each set.

Variations/progressions

- Place a marker dot in one of the squares; here the youngster stops, counts to 3 and starts again
- Place a marker dot in one of the squares; here the youngster repeats the last jump again, i.e. another jump with feet together or a jump with feet across either side
- When the feet come together, stand on one foot; add stability work by holding that position for 5 seconds.

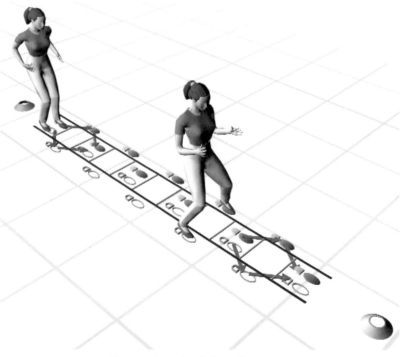

Figure 3.9 Fast foot ladder – hopscotch

DRILL   *FAST FOOT LADDER –*
TWO STEPS FORWARDS AND ONE STEP BACK

Aim
To develop forwards and backwards momentum, balance, stability and control.

Area/equipment
Use an indoor or outdoor area. Use a Fast Foot Ladder – ensure that this is the correct ladder for the type of surface being used.

Description
Youngster to take 2 single steps forwards, one step backwards, and repeat this pattern of movement to the end of the ladder.

Key teaching points
■ Start slowly, build up the speed gradually
■ Ensure arms are correctly used
■ It is important that arms are not swung across the body, as this will throw the youngster off balance
■ Youngster to stand tall and use strong core
■ Arms to be driven while moving forwards *and* backwards.

Sets and reps
2 sets of 3 reps with 1 minute recovery between each set.

Variations/progressions
■ Place a marker dot in a ladder square; when the youngster lands on that square, he or she steps out of the ladder and then back in, then recommences the drill down the ladder
■ Drill can be performed sideways, remember to work both left and right shoulders.

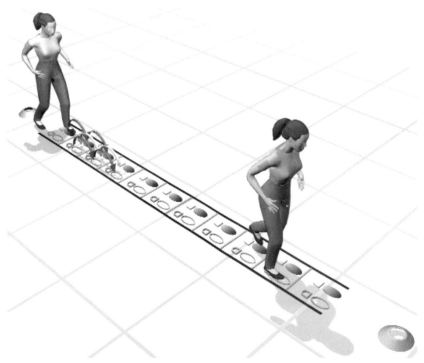

Figure 3.10 Fast foot ladder – two steps forwards and one step back

| DRILL | FAST FOOT LADDER – SINGLE SPACE JUMPS |

Aim

To develop small, controlled jumps with speed, precision, balance and co-ordination.

Area/equipment

Use an indoor or outdoor area. Use a Fast Foot Ladder – ensure that this is the correct ladder for the type of surface being used.

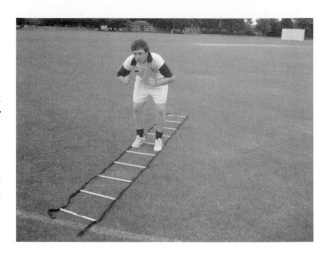

Description

Youngster covers the length of the ladder by jumping into each ladder space with both feet together, and returns to the start by jogging back beside the ladder.

Key teaching points

- Maintain correct jumping form/mechanics
- Start slowly and gradually increase the speed
- Ensure that arms are used in the correct manner to assist the jumps
- Maintain upright posture
- Ensure that on landing youngster does not sink too deep into the hips
- Stress that quality not quantity is important.

Sets and reps

2 sets of 3 reps with 1 minute recovery between each set.

Variations/progressions

- Youngster to throw beanbag into one of the ladder squares; at this square the youngster steps over the beanbag and continues to the end of the ladder
- Place 2 or 3 marker dots into different squares; on landing on the dot the youngster holds the position for 3 to 4 seconds – this is good for developing stability – then continues down the ladder.

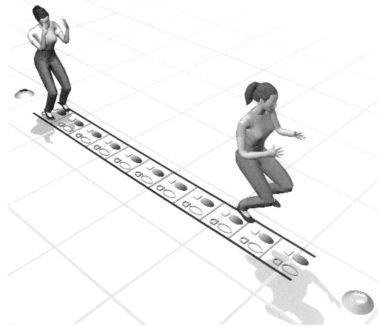

Figure 3.11 Fast foot ladder – single space jumps

DRILL   *FAST FOOT LADDER –*
TWO JUMPS FORWARDS AND ONE JUMP BACK

Aim
To develop forwards and backwards momentum, balance, stability and control while jumping.

Area/equipment
Use an indoor or outdoor area. Use a Fast Foot Ladder – ensure that this is the correct ladder for the type of surface being used.
NB: An outdoor ladder on a hard surface must not be used for this drill.

Description
Youngster takes 2 single jumps forwards, one jump backwards, and repeats this pattern of movement to the end of the ladder.

Key teaching points
- Start slowly, build up the speed gradually
- Land and take off on the balls of the feet
- Ensure arms are correctly used
- Important that arms are not swung across the body; this will throw the youngster off balance
- Youngster to stand tall and use strong core
- Arms to be driven while moving forwards *and* backwards
- Youngsters not to go so fast that they lose control at the end of the ladder.

Sets and reps
2 sets of 3 reps with 1 minute recovery between each set.

Variations/progressions
- Place a marker dot in a ladder square; when the youngster lands on that square, he or she jumps out of the ladder then back in, then recommences the drill down the ladder
- Drill can be performed sideways; remember to work both left and right shoulders.

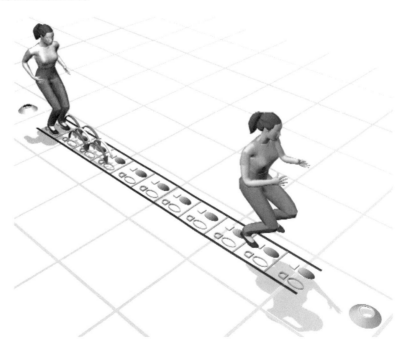

Figure 3.12 Fast foot ladder – two jumps forwards and one jump back

DRILL FAST FOOT LADDER – 'TWIST AGAIN'

Aim
To develop controlled and balanced hip twisting rotation skills.

Area/equipment
Use an indoor or outdoor area. Use a Fast Foot Ladder – ensure that this is the correct ladder for the type of surface being used.

Description
Youngster to move down the ladder with feet together in a twisting movement. Feet to be pointing to the left in one ladder square then pointing to the right when landing in the next square.

Key teaching points
■ Work on the balls of the feet
■ Use arms to help balance
■ Hips to be twisted with control
■ Do not sink into the hips.

Sets and reps
2 sets of 3 reps with 1 minute recovery between each set.

Variations/progressions
■ Perform drill sideways down the ladder
■ Place marker dot in one of the ladder squares; on reaching the dot, youngster to hold position for 3 seconds to help stability, then recommence the drill to the end of the ladder.

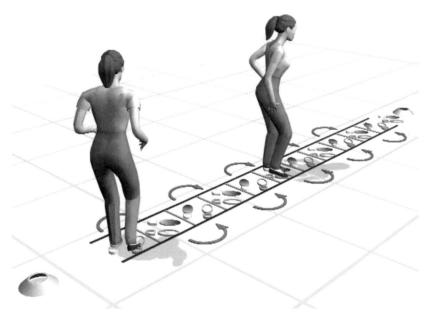

Figure 3.13 Fast foot ladder – 'twist again'

DRILL   *FAST FOOT LADDER – HOP IN-AND-OUT*

Aim
To develop balance, co-ordination and body control.

Area/equipment
Use an indoor or outdoor area. Use a Fast Foot Ladder – ensure that this is the correct ladder for the type of surface being used.

Description
Youngster hops in the ladder square, then out to the side of the next square and back into the ladder square. This sequence is maintained down the ladder. Youngster to perform drill with left leg and then with right leg.

Key teaching points
- Work on the balls of the feet
- Use correct arm mechanics for drive, balance and control
- Do not bend at the hips.

Sets and reps
2 sets of 3 reps with 1 minute recovery between each set.

Variations/progressions
- Introduce hopping from one side of the ladder into a ladder square then out to the other side of the ladder
- Place marker dot in one of the ladder squares; on reaching the dot, youngster to hold position for 3 seconds to help stability, then recommence the drill to the end of the ladder.

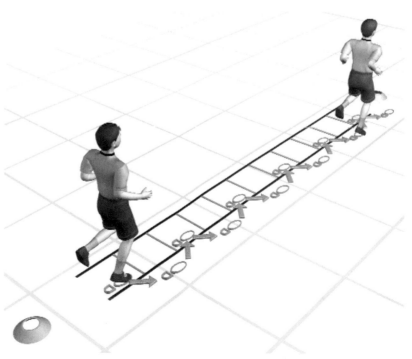

Figure 3.14 Fast foot ladder – hop in and out

DRILL	FAST FOOT LADDER – CARIOCA

Aim
To develop hip mobility and speed, balance and control.

Area/equipment
Use an indoor or outdoor area. Use a Fast Foot Ladder – ensure that this is the correct ladder for the type of surface being used.

Description
Youngster to cover the length of the ladder by moving laterally performing Carioca. The rear foot crosses in front of the body then moves around to the back while, simultaneously, the lead foot does the opposite. The arms also move across the front and back of the body.

Key teaching points
- Start slowly and build up the tempo
- Work on the balls of the feet
- Keep the shoulders square
- Always perform drill on both sides.

Sets and reps
2 sets of 3 reps with 1 minute recovery between each set.

Variation/progression
- Perform the drill with 2 ladders placed next to each other so that the youngsters can complete the drill while mirroring each other.

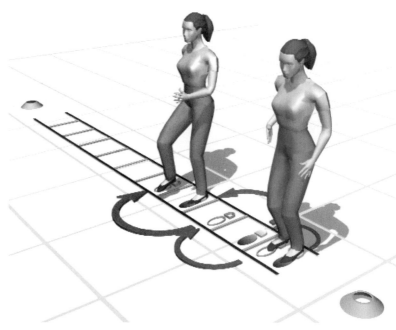

Figure 3.15 Fast foot ladder – carioca

DRILL   *FAST FOOT LADDER – SPOTTY DOGS*

Aim
To improve shoulder and arm speed and activate core muscles. To develop explosive forward and backward stepping movement with co-ordination and balance.

Area/equipment
Use an indoor or outdoor area. Use Fast Food Ladder – ensure that this is the correct ladder for the type of surface being used.

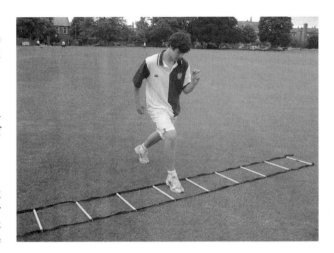

Description
Youngster to cover the length of the ladder moving laterally, alternately stepping in and out of the ladder squares while chopping the legs and arms, left leg to right arm, right leg to left arm. ROM for the arms is from the side of the body up to the side of the face.

Key teaching points
- Keep on the heels
- Arm action is a chop not a punch
- Land and take off on the balls of the feet
- Maintain upright posture
- Keep the head up.

Sets and reps
2 sets of 3 reps with 1 minute recovery between each step.

Variations/progressions
- Youngster can perform the drill using opposite arms and legs
- Youngster can perform the drill holding a beanbag in each hand
- Youngster can perform the drill holding a balloon in each hand.

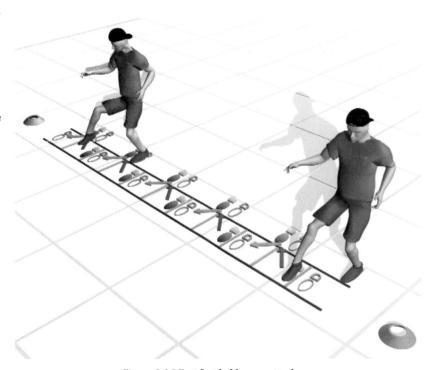

Figure 3.16 Fast foot ladder – spotty dogs

DRILL **FAST FOOT LADDER – T FORMATION**

Aim
To develop linear and lateral change of direction and patterns of movement.

Area/equipment
Use indoor or outdoor area. Place 2 ladders in a T formation with 3 marker dots placed at the end of each ladder.

Description
Youngster accelerates down the ladder using single steps. On reaching the ladder crossing the end, the youngster moves laterally either left or right, using short lateral steps. On coming out of the ladder the youngster then turns and runs back to the start.

Key teaching points
■ Maintain correct running form/mechanics
■ Use strong arm drive when transferring from linear to lateral steps

Sets and reps
3 sets of 4 reps with 1 minute recovery between each set (2 moving to the left and 2 to the right).

Variations/progressions
■ Start with a lateral run and upon reaching the end ladder accelerate in a straight line forwards down the ladder
■ Mix and match previous quick feet ladder drills described earlier.

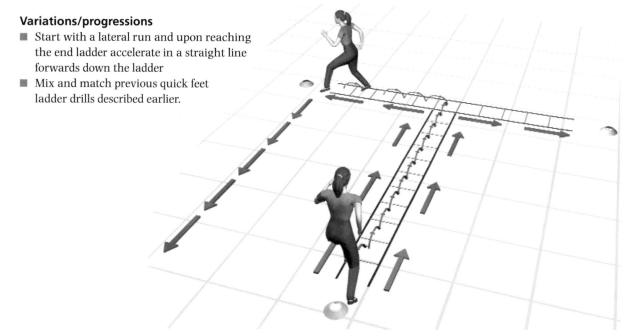

Figure 3.17 Fast foot ladder – T formation

| DRILL | *FAST FOOT LADDER – CROSSOVER* |

Aim
To develop speed, agility and change of direction. To improve youngster's reaction time, peripheral vision and timing.

Area/equipment
Use large indoor or outdoor area. Place 4 ladders in a cross formation leaving a clear centre square of about 3 square yards. Place a marker dot 1 yard from the start of each ladder.

Description
Split the youngsters into 4 equal groups and locate 1 group at the start of each ladder. First youngster from each group accelerates simultaneously down the ladders performing a single-step drill; on reaching the end, youngster accelerates across the centre square and joins the end of the queue for the opposite ladder (without travelling down it).

Key teaching points
- Maintain correct running form/mechanics
- Keep the head and eyes up and be aware of other youngsters, particularly round the centre area.

Sets and reps
3 sets of 6 reps with 1 minute recovery between each set.

Variations/progressions
- At the end of the first ladder, sidestep to the right or left and join the appropriate adjacent ladder
- Vary the Fast Foot Ladder drills performed down the first ladder
- Include a 360-degree turn in the centre square; this is effective for positional awareness.

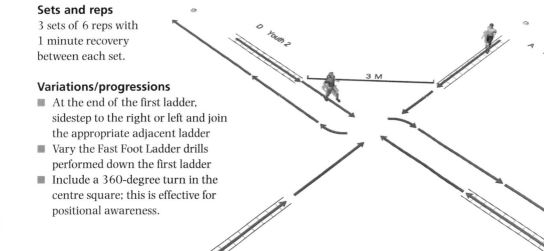

Figure 3.18 Fast foot ladder – crossover

DRILL FAST FOOT LADDER – CROSSOVER HEAD TO HEAD

Aim
To develop linear acceleration, change of direction and visual awareness.

Area/equipment
Use indoor or outdoor area, place 2 ladders in line with a 5-yard gap in the middle. Place a marker spot at the start of each ladder.

Description
Youngsters split up into 2 groups, one group at the start of each ladder. Simultaneously, the youngsters accelerate down the ladder towards each other performing single step drill, then accelerate into the middle space still towards each other. They then swerve and pass each other on the outside, and join the queue at the start of the opposite ladder without travelling down it.

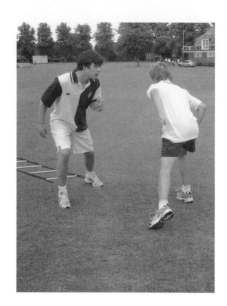

Key teaching points
■ Maintain correct running form
■ Keep eyes and head up and be aware of other youngsters
■ Ensure youngsters are aware of which side they are passing each other in the centre area.

Sets and reps
3 sets of 6 reps, with 1 minute recovery between each set.

Variations/progressions
■ Include 360-degree turn as they come out of the ladder
■ Introduce a beanbag pass in the middle.

DRILL
FAST FOOT LADDER –
MIRROR (FOOT STAMP GAME)

Aim
To develop explosive footwork and footwork reactions.

Area/equipment
Use indoor or outdoor area. Use one 15-foot section of ladder.

Description
Youngster 1 and youngster 2 stand opposite each other on either side of the ladder. Starting in the middle, youngster 1 moves laterally and randomly steps in and out of the ladder. Youngster 2 responds by mirroring as quickly and accurately as possible the movements of youngster 1.

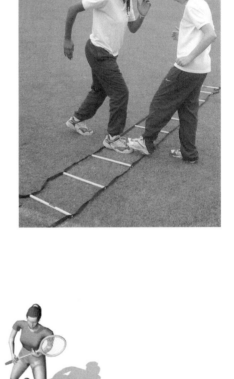

Key teaching points
- Maintain correct lateral running form/mechanics
- Use short, sharp, explosive steps
- Work off the balls of the feet
- Use a strong arm drive
- Always keep the hips square.

Sets and reps
3 sets of 2 reps with 15 seconds rest between reps and 2 minutes recovery between each set. NB: In 1 set each youngster should take the lead for 45 seconds.

Variations/progressions
- Introduce slight upper body, game-like contact
- Introduce racquets, sticks, recreate movements within game situation.

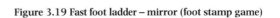

Figure 3.19 Fast foot ladder – mirror (foot stamp game)

DRILL   FAST FEET – LINE DRILLS

Aim
To develop quickness of the feet.

Area/equipment
Indoor or outdoor area. Use any line marked on the ground.

Description
Youngsters perform single split steps over the line and back.

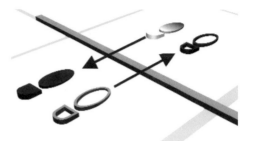

Figure 3.20(a) Fast feet – line drills (split steps)

Key teaching points
■ Maintain good arm mechanics
■ Maintain an upright posture
■ Maintain a strong core
■ Try to develop a rhythm
■ Keep the head and eyes up.

Sets and reps
3 sets of 20 reps with 1 minute recovery between each set.

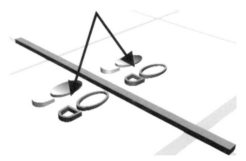

Figure 3.20(b) Two-footed jumps

Variations/progressions
■ Two-footed jumps over the line and back
■ Stand astride the line and bring the feet in to touch the line before moving them out again. Perform the drill as quickly as possible
■ Two-footed side jumps over the line and back
■ Two-footed side jumps with a 180-degree twist in the air over the line and back
■ Single quick hops
■ Complex variation – introduce the ball either at the end of the drill for the youngster to accelerate on to, or during the drill for him or her to pass back before continuing.

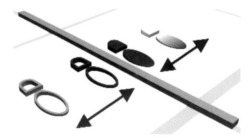

Figure 3.20(c) Standing astride the line

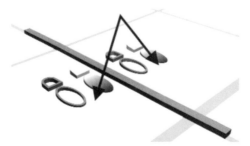

Figure 3.20(d) Two-footed lateral jumps

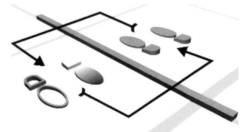

Figure 3.20(e) Two-footed lateral jumps with 180-degree twist

DRILL QUICK BOX STEPS

Aim
To develop explosive power and control. NB: The emphasis is on speed.

Area/equipment
Indoor or outdoor area; a bench, aerobics step or suitable strong box with a non-slip surface, about 12 inches high.

Description
Youngster performs an alternated split step on the box, i.e. one foot on the box and one on the floor.

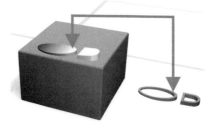

Figure 3.21(a) Split step

Key teaching points
- Focus on good arm drive
- Maintain an upright posture
- Maintain a strong core
- Keep the head/eyes up
- Work off the balls of the feet
- Work at a high intensity level
- Try to develop a rhythm.

Sets and reps
3 sets of 20 reps with 1 minute recovery between each set.

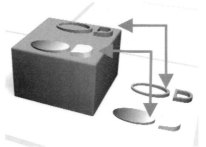

Figure 3.21(b) Two-footed jumps

Variations/progressions
- Two-footed jumps on and off the box
- Two-footed side jumps on and off the box
- Straddle jumps
- Single-footed hops onto the box and off (10 reps leading with the left foot and 10 with the right)
- Alternate single hop – single hop onto the box to land on the opposite foot. Take off to land on the other side of the box, again on the opposite foot.

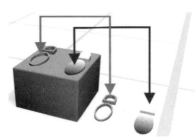

Figure 3.21(c) Two-footed side jumps

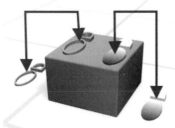

Figure 3.21(d) Straddle jumps

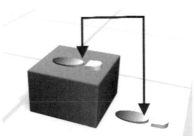

Figure 3.21(e) Single-footed hops

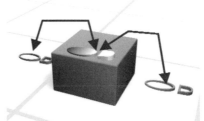

Figure 3.21(f) Alternate single hop

CHAPTER 4 ACCUMULATION OF POTENTIAL

COMBINING QUALITY AND QUICKNESS OF MOVEMENT

In this part of the Youth Continuum we bring together the areas of work already practised. Many of the Dynamic Flex, Mechanics and Innervation practices are specific to developing a particular skill. When youngsters play, exercise and compete in sport a whole range of movements occur which include hand–eye and foot co-ordination, and body and visual awareness. Manipulation skills such as throwing and catching can also be present. An example is a simple game of tag; youngsters will accelerate, decelerate, sidestep, dodge, jump and even step backwards to avoid being caught. These movements happen in a sequence and will occur over a varying period of time. It is here that the full range of Speed, Agility and Quickness can be observed.

Up to this point we have looked at numerous Dynamic Flex, Mechanics and Innervation drills and practices in isolation. This part of the Youth Continuum begins to bring these drills together to combine movements. This is vital for good development because of course when youngsters are physically active through play or sport, movements are clustered not isolated.

Programmed agility circuits are an incredibly effective way of combining movements in a controlled environment. Over a period of time as the youngsters become more competent we can also look to incorporate manipulation skills such as throwing and catching. These in turn will place greater demands on hand–eye and foot co-ordination and work towards developing an all-round athlete. There also exists an excellent opportunity to create an environment that promotes Health Related Fitness and conditioning activity with youngsters.

This section may also be used by the teacher/coach to evaluate youngsters' progress in a structured way.

Health and safety

- Lay out circuits carefully with respect to spacing

- Monitor fatigue levels, allowing appropriate rest periods

- Regarding Agility Discs (where used), no running, jumping or sliding onto/off discs should be permitted.

DRILL AGILITY DISC

Aim
To develop balance, proprioception and stability.

Area/equipment
Use an indoor or outdoor area and an agility disc.

Description
Youngster to stand and balance with both feet on the agility disc.

Key teaching points
- Keep strong core
- Do not sink into the hips
- Use arms to help maintain balance
- Keep head still.

Sets and reps
1 set of 5 reps of 45 seconds, with 15 seconds recovery

Variations/progressions
- Get-ups: Youngster starts in a low position on the agility disc, stands up, and finishes on one leg
- Pass ball to youngster on disc who volleys it back
- Youngster stops a rolling ball
- Youngster catches a passed ball
- Youngster bends and touches a nominated marker spot
- Practise striking skills.

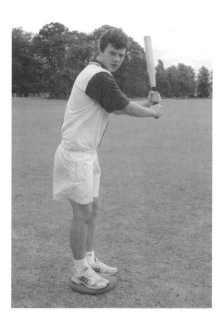

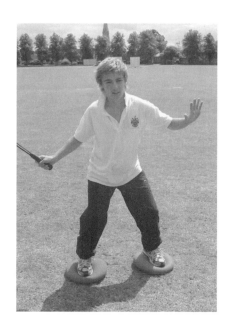

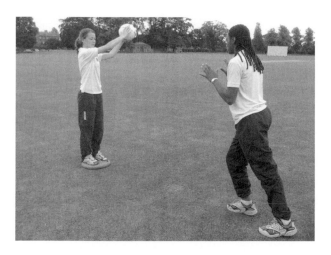

DRILL   *SEATED AGILITY DISC*

Aim
To develop core proprioception, balance and stability.

Area/equipment
Use an indoor or outdoor area and an agility disc.

Description
Youngster sits on agility disc, keeping as upright as possible. Legs are held out slightly bent. First, one foot is raised off the ground and then, when mastered, both feet are raised off the ground together and held for the allotted time.

Key teaching points
- Always start with one foot off the ground first
- Keep head still and up
- Use arms to maintain balance.

Sets and reps
1 set of 5 reps of 45 seconds, with 15 seconds recovery.

Variations/Progressions
- Both feet up
- Pairs back to back, passing the ball around
- 'Simon says' arm movements game
- Pairs, both seated, passing a ball back and forth
- Core stability – throw and catch a jelly ball.

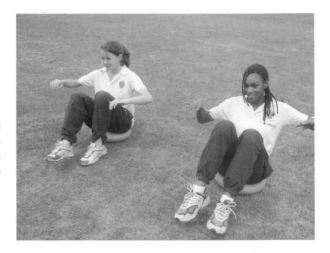

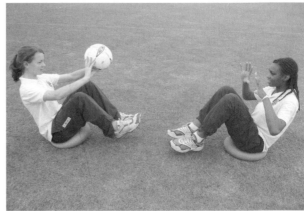

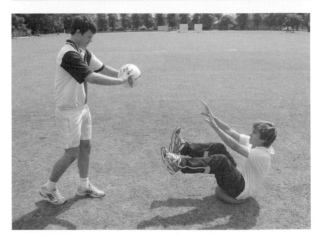

DRILL *SWERVE DEVELOPMENT RUNS*

Aim

To develop fine-angled swerve running, balance, co-ordination and body control.

Area/equipment

Use a large indoor or outdoor area. Place 8–12 poles, cones or marker spots in a zigzag formation. The distance between them should be 1½–2 yards at varying angles (this will make the runs more realistic). The total length of the run will be 15–20 yards.

Description

The youngster accelerates from the first cone and swerves from inside the channel turning from cone to cone, then gently jogs back to the starting cone before repeating the drill.

Key teaching points

- Maintain correct running form/mechanics
- Work on shortening the steps used in the turn
- Focus on increasing the speed of the arm drive when coming out of the turns
- Take tight, not wide, angles around the cones
- Keep the head and eyes up.

Sets and reps

2 sets of 3 reps, with 30 seconds recovery between each rep and 1 minute recovery between each set.

Variation/Progression

Go around the cones.

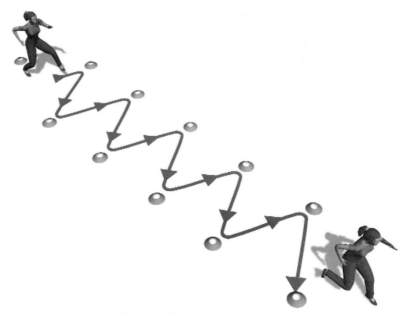

Figure 4.1 Swerve development runs

DRILL   FAST FEET ZIGZAG RUNS

Aim
To develop acceleration, transfer from linear to lateral zigzag movement back to linear movement with control, balance and precision.

Area/equipment
Use an indoor or outdoor area, mark out a grid using 2 ladders and 10 to 12 cones or poles; place ladder first then the cones or poles in a zigzag formation finally finishing off with a ladder at the end (see fig. 4.2).

Description
Youngster runs down the ladder to develop acceleration; on leaving the ladder the youngster moves sideways to the first cone and repeats this movement up to the last cone. On the last cone the youngster straightens up and runs down the final ladder, then walks back to the start and repeats the drill.

Key teaching points
- Maintain correct running form/mechanics
- Hips must face forwards and not be twisted
- Use short steps
- Do not skip
- Use good arm mechanics

NB: Arm mechanics are as vital in lateral movements as they are in linear movements; many youngsters forget to use their arms when they are moving sideways.

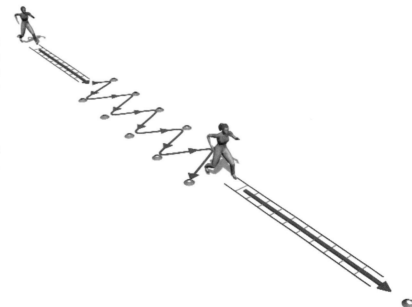

Sets and reps
2 sets of 3 reps with a walk-back recovery between each rep and 1 minute recovery between each set.

Variations/progressions
- Vary the drills on the ladder
- Up-and-back – enter the grid sideways and move forwards to the first cone then backwards to the next.

Figure 4.2 Fast feet zigzag runs

DRILL   FOUR TURN, FOUR ANGLE RUN

Aim

To develop turns and angled change of direction with control, balance and co-ordination.

Area/equipment

Use indoor or outdoor area, using 5 marker dots, cones or poles placed in a cross formation with a centre cone. The points of the cross are equally spaced out 5 yards from the centre.

Description

Youngster starts on the centre cone E, and runs around cone A and back to the centre cone E, changes angle of the run to move out towards and around cone B, and then back to the centre cone E. This is continued for cones C and D.

Sets and reps

2 sets of 2 reps with 1 minute recovery between each set and 2 minutes between each rep.

Variation/Progression

Add 2 or 3 additional cones between centre cone E and cones B and D. Here the youngster swerves in between the cones, out and back.

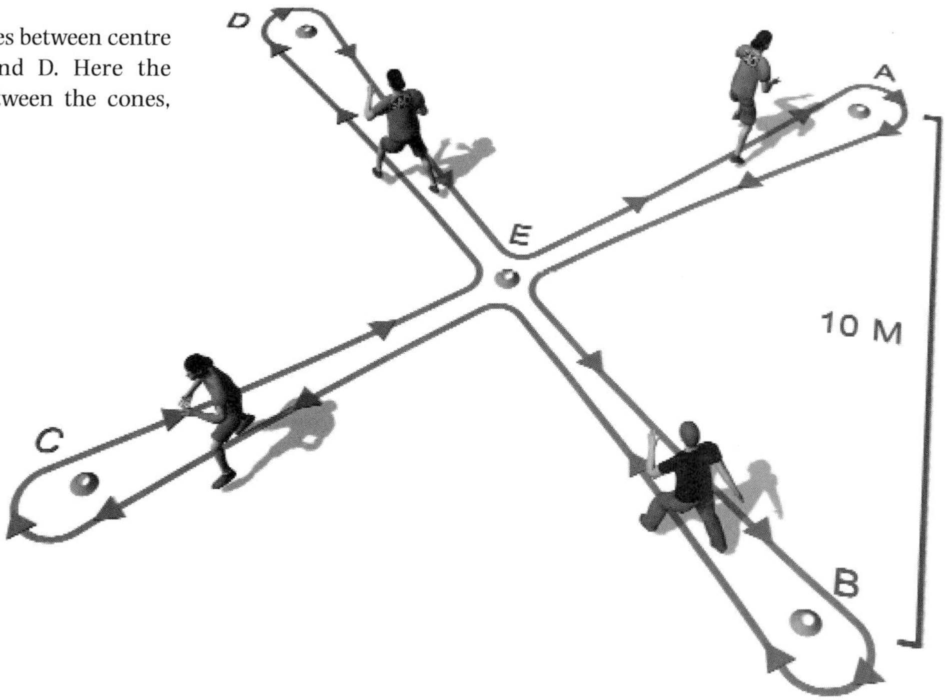

Figure 4.3 Four turn, four angle run

DRILL   COMBINATION RUNS

Aim

To develop a combination of running and movement patterns that will help develop the youngster's gross motor skills.

Area/equipment

Indoor or outdoor area, depending on size of the space available. Place hurdles, fast foot ladder, poles/cones/marker dots in different formations and combinations.

Description

Youngster to complete circuit performing the different drills, i.e. stepping, jumping, swerving etc.

Key teaching point

Maintain correct running form/mechanics for all activities.

Sets and reps

2 sets of 2 reps with 1 minute recovery between each set and 2 minutes recovery between each rep.

Variations/progressions

- Vary the drills at hurdles, ladders etc.
- Set out identical circuits and introduce team relays.

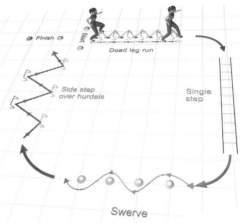

Figure 4.4(a) Combination run 1

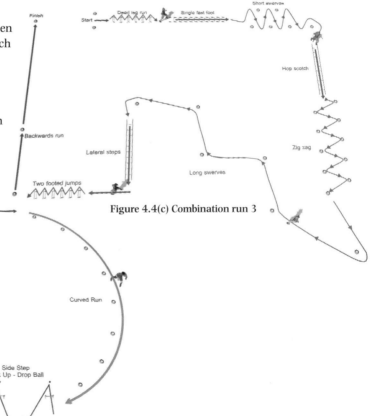

Figure 4.4(c) Combination run 3

Figure 4.4(b) Combination run 2

DRILL *TEAM COMBINATION RUNS*

Aim

To develop multidirectional movement, balance, co-ordination and body control while competing against another team.

Area/equipment

Use a large indoor or outdoor area, depending on size of the space available. Place 2 sets of identical hurdles, Fast Foot Ladder, poles/cones/marker dots in different formations and combinations next to each other. Ensure there is a starting and finishing point for the teams.

Description

Teams to complete circuit performing the different drills, i.e. stepping, jumping, swerving etc, while competing against the other team. The team that finishes first or has fewest mistakes is the winner.

Key teaching points

- Maintain correct running form/mechanics for all activities
- Ensure that speed is not sacrificed for quality of movement.

Sets and reps

2 sets of 2 reps with 1 minute recovery between each set and 2 minutes recovery between each rep.

Variations/progressions

- Vary the drills at hurdles, ladders etc.
- Set out identical circuits and introduce team relays.

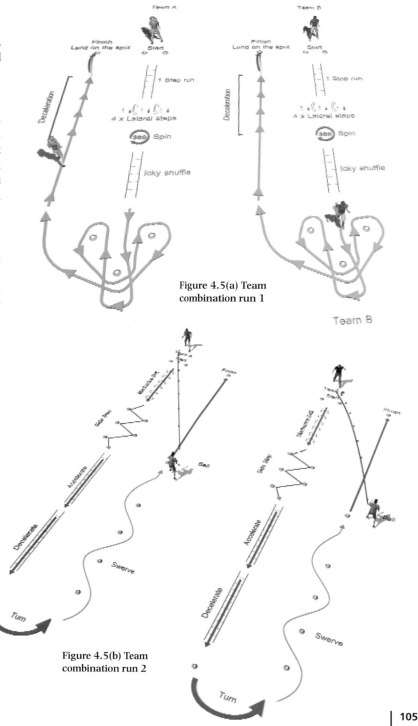

Figure 4.5(a) Team combination run 1

Figure 4.5(b) Team combination run 2

DRILL   HEALTH-RELATED FITNESS CIRCUITS

Aim

To improve general health and fitness including cardiovascular health, balance, agility, co-ordination, reactions, manipulation and visual skills; to be challenged and to have fun at the same time.

Area/equipment

Use an indoor or outdoor area with marker spots, hurdles, ladders, mats, agility disc and jelly balls or tennis balls or beanbags. Equipment to be set out in stations so that different drills can be performed.

Description

Youngsters to perform drills at each station for an allotted time, then move to the next station in the circuit to perform the next drill.

Key teaching points

- Use the correct techniques required for each station, i.e. correct arm mechanics, posture etc.
- Ensure that all drills are demonstrated prior to warming up
- Provide constant feedback to all youngsters during circuit.

Sets and reps

1 circuit, 40 seconds per station with a 25-second change-over.

Variation/progression

Add different drills at each station.

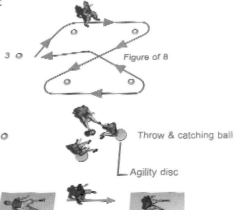

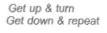

Figure 4.6 Health-related fitness circuit

CHAPTER 5 EXPLOSION

IMPROVING THE CONTROL AND QUICKNESS OF RESPONSE

All youngsters have the ability to improve response times and develop multidirectional explosive movements. While helping youngsters to understand, for example, that getting to the ball/space first is essential in games play it is possible to develop their ability to move explosively both in a horizontal and vertical direction. 'Let go' and 'get-up' drills all develop the abilities for youngsters to be more explosive. The most crucial element of using these types of drill is the implementation of the contrast phase. This simply means performing a drill without resistance for one or two reps, directly after performing them with resistance. An example of this is running with a Sonic Chute twice over 20 yards and running again without.

The key is to ensure that quality not quantity is the priority, and efforts must be carefully monitored. This is a time for fast action, not exhausting, tongue-hanging-out responses and fatigue.

Health and safety

- Monitor quantities of effort
- Create clear working grids to avoid collisions
- Always follow lesson application guidelines and any equipment instructions
- Allow for plenty of 'run-out space', i.e. not too close to walls.

DRILL　　VISION AND REACTION – FAST HAND GAMES

Aim
To develop lightning-quick hand–eye reactions; to be both fun and challenging.

Area/equipment
Indoor or outdoor area. No equipment required.

Description
Working in pairs, youngster1 puts his or her hands together and holds them slightly away in front of the chest. Youngster 2 stands directly in front with hands held at the side. The drill begins with youngster 2 attempting to slap youngster 1's hands. Youngster 1 tries to prevent youngster 2 by moving the hands away as quickly as possible. Youngsters alternate.

Key teaching points
- Stand in athletic position
- Keep head still.

Sets and reps
30 seconds each per drill.

Variations/progressions
- Youngster 1 holds his or her hands out with the palms facing the ground, with tips of thumbs just touching. Youngster 2 holds hands just above. The drill commences with youngster 2 attempting to slap both hands before youngster 1 can react by moving them away
- Youngster 1 stands directly in front of youngster 2, 1 or 2 yards away. Youngster 1 jabs a punch at youngster 2 who attempts to clap both hands over the fist.

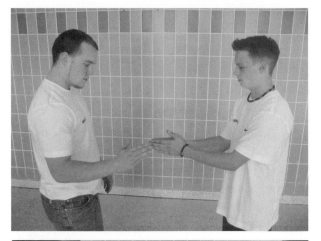
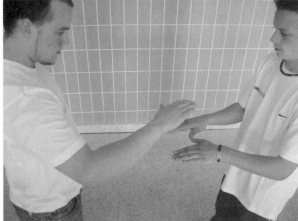
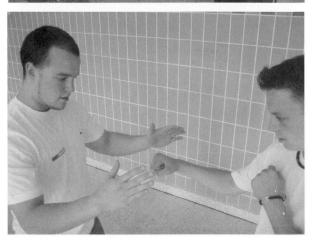

DRILL | *VISION AND REACTION - REACTION BALL*

Aim
To develop lightning-quick hand–eye reactions.

Area/equipment
Outdoor or indoor area but not a grass surface. Use 1 Reaction Ball or a tennis/foam ball or beanbag.

Description
Work in pairs or small groups; standing 5 yards apart. The ball/beanbag is thrown so that it lands in front of the youngster, because of the structure of the ball it will bounce in any direction. The youngster has to react and catch the ball before it bounces for a second time.

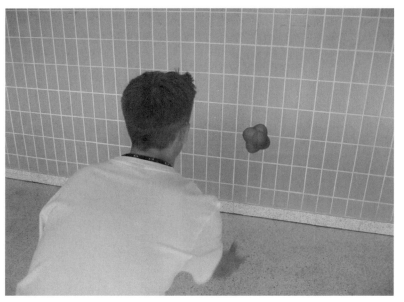

Key teaching points
■ The youngster catching the ball should work off the balls of the feet and in a slightly crouched position with the hands out ready
■ The ball/beanbag should not be thrown hard – it will do the necessary work itself.

Sets and reps
2 set of 20 reps with no recovery between each rep and 1 minute recovery between each set.

Variations/progressions
■ Work individually or in pairs by throwing the ball/beanbag against the wall
■ Stand on agility discs while throwing the ball/beanbag to each other.

DRILL   *GET-UPS*

Aim
To develop multidirectional explosive acceleration. To improve a youngster's ability to get up and accelerate all in one movement.

Area/equipment
Indoor or outdoor area of 10 square yards.

Description
Youngster sits on the floor, facing the direction she or he is going to run in with her or his legs straight out in front. On the signal from the teacher/coach, the youngster gets up as quickly as possible, accelerates for 5 yards and then slows down before jogging gently back to the start position.

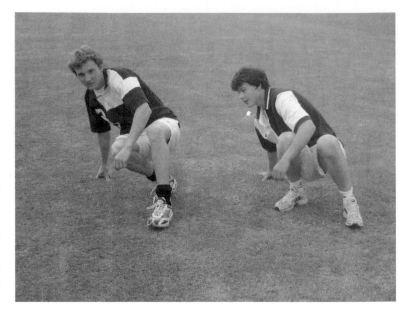

Key teaching points
■ Try to complete the drill in one smooth action
■ Use correct running form/mechanics
■ Do not stop between getting up and starting to run
■ Get into an upright position and drive the arms as soon as possible
■ Ensure the initial steps are short and powerful
■ Do not overstride.

Sets and reps
2 sets of 4 reps with a jog-back recovery between each rep and 2 minutes recovery between each set.

Variations/progressions
■ Backward get-ups
■ Sideways get-ups
■ Lying get-ups from the front, back, left and right
■ Kneeling get-ups
■ Work in pairs and have get-up competitions chasing the ball
■ Work in pairs with one youngster in front of the other and perform 'tag' get-ups.

DRILL *CHAIR GET-UPS*

Aim
To develop explosive power for acceleration linearly and laterally.

Area/equipment
Indoor or outdoor area with plenty of room for deceleration – place a chair or stool and 5 markers as shown below.

Description
Youngster sits on a chair, and on the teacher/coach's signal will get up and move to the nominated marker dot/cone as quickly as possible. On reaching the marker dot/cone the youngster should decelerate and walk back to the start position.

Key teaching points
- Use an explosive arm drive when getting up
- Get into a correct running posture as quickly as possible
- Initial steps should be short and powerful
- Work off the balls of the feet.

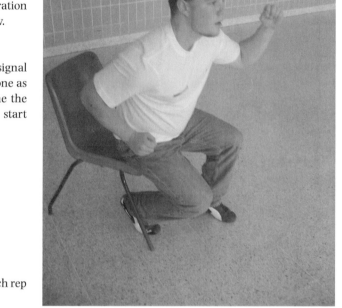

Sets and reps
2 sets of 6 reps with a walk-back recovery between each rep and 2 minutes recovery between each set.

Variation/progression
Introduce a 1:2 passing drill at the cones/marker dots.

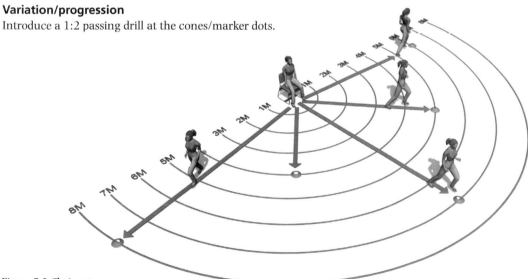

Figure 5.1 Chair get-ups

DRILL | *LET-GOES*

Aim
To develop multidirectional explosive acceleration.

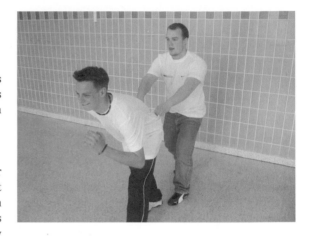

Area/equipment
Indoor or outdoor area of 10 square yards; ensure there is plenty of room for safe deceleration. NB: strong clothing is preferred; if youngsters are wearing light clothing then a towel can be used.

Description
Working in pairs, youngster 1 stands directly in front of her or his partner, youngster 2, and grips her or his shorts or shirt on both sides. Youngster 1 tries to accelerate away from youngster 2, who resists the movement for a few seconds before releasing youngster 1. Youngster 1 accelerates away for 2–4 yards before decelerating and walking back to the start position.

Key teaching points
- Work off the balls of the feet
- Use short steps during the explosion and acceleration phases
- Use good arm drive
- Keep head up
- Youngster 1 should adopt good running form/mechanics as soon as possible.

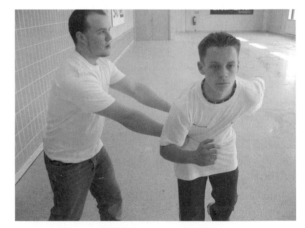

Sets and reps
2 sets of 3 reps with a walk-back recovery between each rep and 2 minutes recovery between each set.

Variations/progressions
- Lateral let-goes
- Backward let-goes
- Let-goes with an acceleration onto a stationary ball
- Let-goes with an acceleration onto a moving ball.

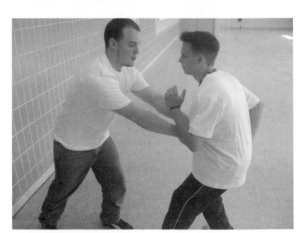

DRILL *PARACHUTE RUNNING*

Aim
To develop explosive running over longer distances (sprint endurance) and explosive acceleration.

Area/equipment
Indoor or outdoor area, 4 marker dots and a parachute. Mark out a grid of 25 yards in length, place one marker dot down as a start marker, and 3 further marker dots at distances of 15, 20 and 25 yards from the start marker.

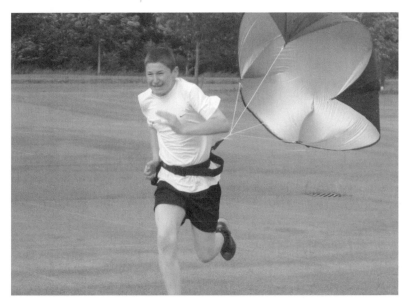

Description
Wearing the parachute, youngster accelerates to the 20-yard marker dot then decelerates.

Key teaching points
- Maintain correct running form/mechanics
- Do not worry if the wind and the resistance cause you to feel as though you are being pulled from side to side; this will in fact improve your balance and co-ordination
- Do not lean into the run too much
- Quality, not quantity, is vital.

Sets and reps
2 sets of 4 reps plus 1 contrast run with a walk-back recovery between each rep and 3 minutes recovery between each set.

Variations/progressions
- Explosive reacceleration – the parachutes have a release mechanism; the youngster accelerates to the 15-yard marker dot where he or she releases the parachute and explodes to the 20-yard marker dot before decelerating
- Random change of direction – the teacher/coach stands behind the 15-yard marker dot; as the youngster releases the parachute the teacher/coach indicates a change in the direction of the run. When mastered, the teacher/coach can then introduce a ball for youngster to run on to during the explosive phase.

DRILL   BALL DROPS

Aim
To develop explosive reactions.

Area/equipment
Indoor or outdoor area; 1 or 2 foam balls

Description
Work in pairs; one youngster drops the ball at various distances and angles from his or her partner. The ball is dropped from shoulder height and immediately the partner explodes forwards and attempts to catch the ball before the second bounce. (Distances between youngsters will differ because the height of the bounce will vary depending on the ground surface.)

Key teaching points
■ Work off the balls of the feet, particularly prior to the drop
■ Use a very explosive arm drive
■ The initial steps should be short, fast and explosive
■ At the take-off do not jump, dither or hesitate
■ Work on developing a smooth one-movement run

Sets and reps
3 sets of 8 reps with 2 minutes recovery between each set.

Variations/progressions
■ Youngster to hold 2 balls and to drop just 1
■ Youngster to hold 2 balls, second youngster has back to him or her. First youngster calls and drops the ball, second youngster turns and accelerates to get to the ball before the second bounce
■ Youngster stands side on to the balls before they are dropped
■ Work in groups of 3 with 2 of the youngsters at different angles alternately dropping a ball for the third youngster to catch; on achieving this, the youngster turns and accelerates away to catch/dive on the second ball. Alter the start positions, e.g. sideways, backwards with a call, seated, etc

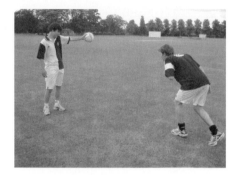

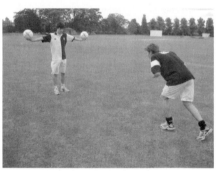

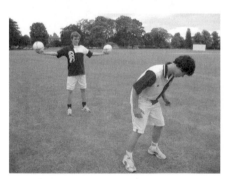

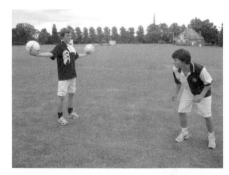

DRILL BUGGY RUNS

Aim
To develop multidirectional explosive acceleration.

Area/equipment
Indoor or outdoor area – ensure that there is plenty of room for safe deceleration. One Viper Belt with a flexi-cord attached at both ends by 2 anchor points. Place 3 markers in a line, 10 yards apart.

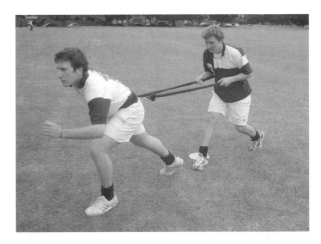

Description
Work in pairs: youngster 1 wears the belt while youngster 2 stands behind holding the flexi-cord, hands looped in and over the cord (for safety purposes). Youngster 2 allows resistance to develop as youngster 1 accelerates forward, then runs behind maintaining constant resistance over the first 10 yards. Both youngsters need to decelerate over the second 10 yards. Youngster 1 removes the belt after the required number of reps and completes a solo contrast run. Repeat the drill but swap roles.

Key teaching points
- Youngster 1 must focus on correct running form/mechanics and explosive drive
- Youngster 2 works with youngster 1, allowing the flexi-cord to provide the resistance.

Sets and reps
1 set of 6 reps plus 1 contrast run with 30 seconds recovery between each rep and 3 minutes recovery before the next exercise.

Variation/progressions
- Lateral buggy run – youngster 1 accelerates laterally for the first 2 yards before turning to cover the remaining distance linearly
- Youngster 2 to throw ball over youngster 1, who reacts and accelerates under resistance and fields the ball.

DRILL   FLEXI-CORD – OUT AND BACK

Aim

To develop short, explosive, angled accelerated runs – ideal for close fielding development.

Area/equipment

Large indoor or outdoor area of 10 square yards would be ideal. Viper Belt with a Flexi-cord attached to 1 anchor point on the belt and a safety belt on the other end of the Flexi-cord. Markers are set out as shown in fig.5.2.

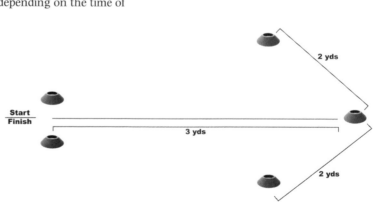

Description

Work in pairs. Youngster 1 wears the Viper Belt, youngster 2 stands directly behind youngster 1 holding the Flexi-cord and wearing the safety belt. The Flexi-cord should be taut at this stage. Youngster 2 nominates a marker for youngster 1, varying between the 3 markers for the required number of repetitions. Youngster 1 runs to the nominated marker, then returns to the start using short, sharp steps. Finish with a contrast run before swapping roles.

Key teaching points

- Focus on short, sharp explosive steps and a fast, powerful arm drive
- Maintain correct running form/mechanics
- Work off the balls of the feet
- Use short steps while returning to the start, and keep the weight forward.

Sets and reps

3 sets of 6 reps plus 1 contrast run per set with 3 minutes recovery between each set. For advanced youngsters, depending on the time of the season, increase to 10 reps.

Variations/progressions

- Perform the drill laterally
- Work backwards with short, sharp steps
- A third youngster or teacher/coach throws a ball to youngster1 to catch and return as they reach the designated marker.

Figure 5.2 Flexi-cord – out and back

DRILL *FLEXI-CORD – OVERSPEED*

Aim
To develop lightning-quick acceleration.

Area/equipment
Indoor or outdoor area; 4 markers and 1 Viper Belt with a Flexi-cord. Place the markers 3 yards apart in a T formation.

Description
Work in pairs. Youngster 1 wears the Viper Belt and faces youngster 2, who holds the Flexi-cord and has the safety belt around his/her waist, i.e. the Flexi-cord will go from belly button to belly button. Youngster 1 stands at marker A, youngster 2 stands at marker B and walks backwards away from youngster 1, thereby increasing the cord's resistance. After stretching the cord for 4–5 yards, youngster 1 accelerates towards youngster 2 who then nominates marker C or D, requiring youngster 1 to change direction explosively. Walk back to the start and repeat the drill.

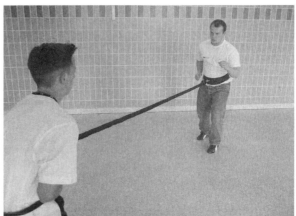

Key teaching points
■ Maintain correct running form/mechanics
■ Control the running form/mechanics
■ During the change of direction phase, shorten the steps and increase the rate of firing of the arms.

Sets and reps
3 sets of 8 reps plus 1 contrast run with 3 minutes recovery between each set.

Variations/progressions
■ Youngster 1 starts with a horizontal jump before accelerating away
■ Introduce a ball which is thrown for youngster 1 to catch after the change of direction phase.

DRILL ASSISTED/RESISTED TOW RUNS

Aim
To develop explosive acceleration and running technique.

Area/equipment
Indoor or outdoor area; 2 Viper Belts joined by 1 Flexi-cord (use 2 Flexi-cords for heavier and stronger youngsters); marker spots.

Description
Youngsters 1 and 2 are attached to one another by the Viper Belt. Youngster 1 runs away from youngster 2 who stands still until pulled forward. Youngster 1 accelerates for 10 yards then decelerates for 5 yards and reaccelerates for another 10 yards. Youngster 2 will accelerate, decelerate then reaccelerate in co-operation with youngster 1. Turn and then repeat on the way back.

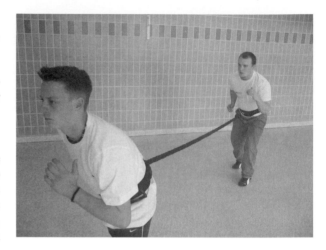

Key teaching points
■ Maintain correct running form and mechanics
■ Both youngsters should use strong arm drive.
■ Both youngsters should use short steps during the acceleration phase
■ Youngster 1 must keep an upwards and forwards lean and not try to resist the acceleration by leaning backwards.

Sets and reps
1 set of 4 reps (1 rep equals once out and back) with a 30 second recovery between each rep.

Variations/Progressions
■ Perform tow runs while swerving round marker spots
■ Youngster to be pulled forward to start facing sideways or backwards, then turn to accelerate.

DRILL

FLEXI-CORD – LATERAL EXPLOSIVE
FIRST STEP DEVELOPMENT

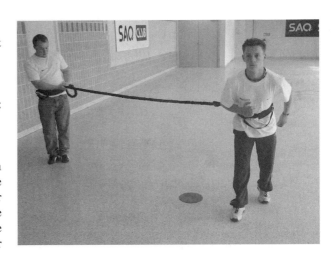

Aim
To develop explosive lateral acceleration – ideal for most sports that require multidirectional, fast first few steps.

Area/equipment
Indoor or outdoor area; Viper Belt; Flexi-cords, foam balls; 12 markers set up as shown in fig. 5.3.

Description
Youngster 1, wearing the Viper Belt, runs a zigzag pattern between the markers. Youngster 2 works along the line between the 2 outside markers slightly behind his or her partner, to ensure that the flexi-cord does not get in the way of the arm mechanics. Work up and back along the line of zigzag markers. On completing the reps, youngster 1 removes the belt and performs 1 contrast run.

Key teaching points
- Maintain correct running form/mechanics
- Use good technique for catching and throwing
- Use short steps going backwards
- Keep the hips square
- Youngster 2 to move along with youngster1, concentrating on maintaining a constant distance, angle and resistance.

Sets and reps
3 sets of 8 reps plus 2 contrast runs and passes with 3 minutes recovery between each set.

Variations/progressions
- Introduce third youngster or teacher/coach who throws the ball to youngster 1 during the drill
- Drill can be performed sideways.

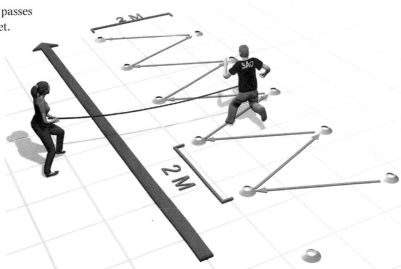

Figure 5.3 Flexi-cord – lateral explosive first step development

DRILL   SIDE-STEPPER – RESISTED LATERAL RUNS

Aim
To develop explosive, controlled lateral patterns of running.

Area/equipment
Indoor or outdoor are; Side-Stepper. Place 10–12 markers in a zigzag pattern.

Description
The youngster wearing the Side-Stepper runs in a lateral zigzag between the markers, down the length of the grid and, just before a marker, extends the last step to increase the level of resistance; then turns round and works back along the grid.

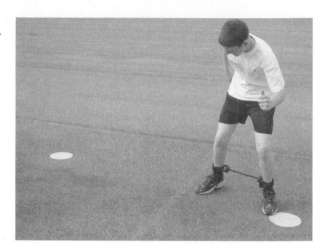

Key teaching points
- Maintain correct lateral running form/mechanics
- Do not sink into the hips when stepping off to change directions
- During the directional change phase, increase arm speed to provide additional control.

Sets and reps
3 sets of 6 reps plus 1 contrast run with 3 minutes recovery between each set.

Variations/progressions
- Perform the drill backwards
- Introduce a foam ball on the change of direction phase.

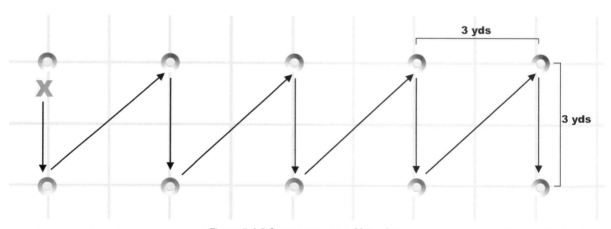

Figure 5.4 Side-stepper – resisted lateral runs

DRILL SIDE-STEPPER – JOCKEYING THROW AND CATCH DRILL

Aim

To develop explosive, lateral/angled movement used in fielding.

Area/equipment

Indoor or outdoor area; 6–8 markers outline a channel about 20 yards long and 3 yards wide; Side-Steppers.

Description

Both youngsters wear a Side-Stepper and face each other about 4 yards apart. Youngster 1 moves from right to left in a backwards pattern while youngster 2 attempts to mirror the movements of youngster 1. The ball is transferred between them throughout the drill. On reaching the end of the grid the roles are now reversed, with youngster 1 moving forwards and youngster 2 moving backwards.

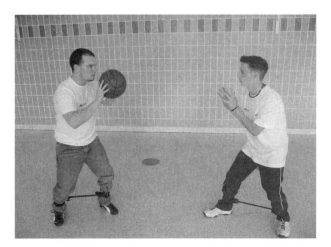

Key teaching points

- Use quick, low steps, *not* high knees
- Do not skip or jump – one foot should be in contact with floor at all times
- Try to keep the feet shoulder-width apart
- Use a powerful arm drive
- Do not sink into the hips.

Sets and reps

3 sets of 4 reps with 30 seconds recovery between each rep and 2 minutes recovery between each set. Youngsters to swap roles after each rep.

Variations/progressions

- Both youngsters perform the drill laterally, one youngster leading and the other trying to mirror
- Youngsters to perform drill with one following the other at the same distance apart. The youngster who is following calls the front youngster to turn and throws him or her the ball to catch, then the drill is reversed.

DRILL HAND-WEIGHT DROPS

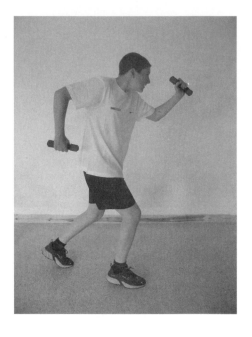

Aim
To develop explosive power, reacceleration and, specifically, a powerful arm drive.

Area/equipment
Indoor or outdoor area; hand weights (2–4 lb). Position 1 marker to mark the start, a second 15 yards away and a final marker 10 yards away from the second.

Description
Youngster with the weights in her or his hands accelerates to the second marker where she or he releases the hand weights, keeping a natural flow to the arm mechanics, then continues to accelerate to the third marker before decelerating and walking back to the start and repeating the drill.

Key teaching points
- Maintain correct running form/mechanics
- Do not stop the arm drive to release the weights
- Keep the head tall
- Quality not quantity is vital.

Sets and reps
3 sets of 4 reps with 3 minutes recovery between each set.

Variations/progressions
- On the release of the hand weights the teacher/coach can call a change of direction – i.e. the youngster is to accelerate off at different angles
- Perform the drill backwards over the first 15 yards then turn, accelerate and release the weights to explode away
- Perform the drill laterally over the first 15 yards then turn, accelerate and release the weights to explode away
- On the release on the hand weights the ball is thrown for the youngster to accelerate and catch.

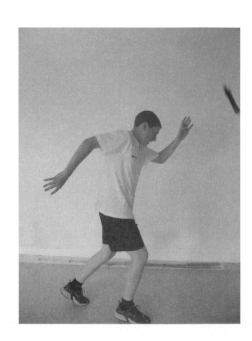

DRILL **BREAK-AWAY MIRROR DRILLS**

Aim
To develop multidirectional explosive reactions.

Area/equipment
Indoor or outdoor area; 1 Break-Away Belt.

Description
Work in pairs, and face each other attached by the Break-Away Belt. Set a time limit. Youngster 1 is proactive while youngster 2 is reactive. Youngster 1 attempts to get away from youngster 2 by using either sideways, forwards or backwards movements; it is not allowed to turn round and run away. The drill ends if and when the proactive youngster breaks the belt connection or the time runs out.

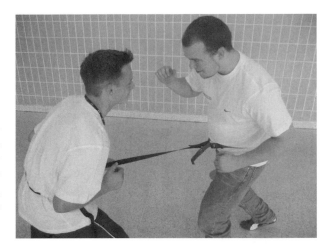

Key teaching points
- Stay focused on your partner
- Do not sink into the hips
- Keep the head tall and the spine straight
- Maintain correct arm mechanics.

Sets and reps
3 sets where 1 set is 30 seconds of each youngster taking the proactive role followed by a 1 minute recovery period.

Variation/progression
- Side-by-side mirror drills - the object is for the proactive youngster to move away laterally and gain as much distance as possible before the other can react.

DRILL MEDICINE BALL (JELLY BALL) WORKOUT

Aim
To develop explosive upper-body and core power.

Area/equipment
Indoor or outdoor area; jelly balls of various weights can be used.

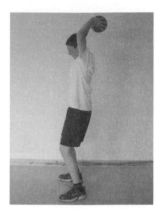
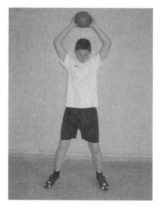

Description
Working in pairs or individually against a wall, the youngsters perform simple throws, e.g. chest passes, single arm passes, front slams, back slams, twist passes, woodchopper and granny throws.

Key teaching points
- Start with a lighter ball for a warm-up set
- Start with simple movements first before progressing to twists etc.
- Keep the spine upright
- Take care when loading (catching) and unloading (throwing) as this can put stress on the lower back.

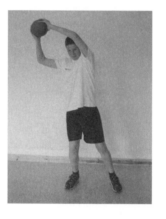
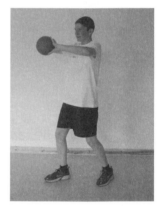

Sets and reps
1 set of 12 reps of each drill with 1 minute recovery between each drill and 3 minutes recovery before the next exercise.

Variations/progressions
- Front slam
- Back slam
- Woodchopper
- Chest pass
- Single arm thrust
- Side slam.

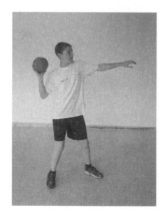
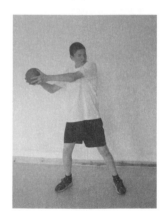

DRILL *PLYOMETRICS – LOW-IMPACT QUICK JUMPS*

Aim
To develop explosive power for running, jumping and changing direction.

Area/equipment
Indoor or outdoor area; Fast Foot Ladder or markers placed 18 inches apart.

Description
The youngster performs double-footed single jumps, i.e. 1 jump between each rung. On reaching the end of the ladder, he or she turns round and jumps back.

Key teaching points
- Maintain correct jumping form/mechanics
- The emphasis is on the speed of the jumps, but do not lose control, i.e. avoid feeling as though you are about to fall over the edge of a cliff when you reach the end of the drill
- Do not lean forwards too much.

Sets and reps
2 sets of 2 reps with 1minute recovery between each set.

Variations/progressions
- Backwards jump
- Two jumps forward and one back
- Sideways jumps
- Sideways jumps, two forwards and one back
- Hopscotch – 2 feet in the square and then 1 foot either side of the next square
- Left-and right-footed hops
- Increase the intensity – replace ladders or markers with 7- or 12-inch hurdles and perform the drills above.

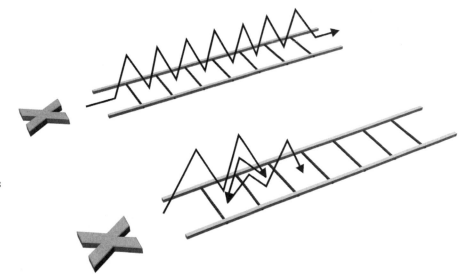

Figure 5.5 Plyometrics – low-impact quick jumps

DRILL   PLYOMETRIC CIRCUIT

Aim
To develop explosive multidirectional speed, agility and quickness.

Area/equipment
Indoor or outdoor area. Place ladders, hurdles and markers in a circuit formation.

Description
Youngsters are to jump, hop and zigzag their way through the circuit as stipulated by the teacher/coach.

Key teaching points
- Maintain the correct mechanics for each part of the circuit
- Ensure that there is a smooth transfer from running to jumping movements and vice versa.

Sets and reps
5 circuits with 1 minute recovery between each circuit.

Variation/progression
Work in pairs. Youngster 1 completes the circuit while youngster 2 feeds the ball at various points around the circuit for youngster 1 to pass back.

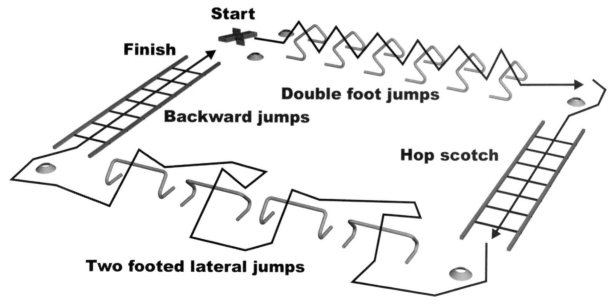

Start

Finish

Double foot jumps

Backward jumps

Hop scotch

Two footed lateral jumps

Figure 5.6 Plyometric circuit

DRILL RESISTED KICKING

Aim
To increase speed and power of foot while striking a ball.

Area/equipment
Indoor or outdoor area; punch kick resistor; ball.

Description
Working in pairs, the punch kick resistor is attached to the ankle of the youngster who is going to perform the kicking drill. His or her partner will hold the other end of the punch kick resistor using the wrap-around handle. The drill is performed with the punch kick resistor stretched so that it provides enough resistance for a back swing and a follow-through of the leg and foot. The youngster starts the drill by taking a normal swing and kick of the ball; this is repeated for the required amount of reps. The punch kick resistor is removed and the ball is kicked without the resistance (contrast phase).

Key teaching points
- Maintain correct kicking technique as much as possible
- Partner to work behind with punch kick resistor so that it does not interfere with the natural swing
- Maintain rhythm and focus on the ball as much as possible
- Do not sink into the hips
- Practise on both legs.

Sets and reps
2 sets of 6 reps with 1 contrast and 2 minutes recovery between each set.

Variation/progression
Perform the drill but attach the punch kick resistor to the wrist for throwing.

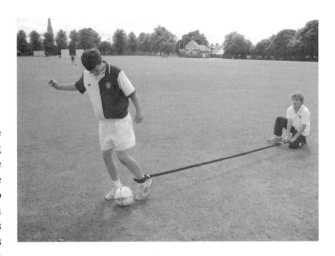

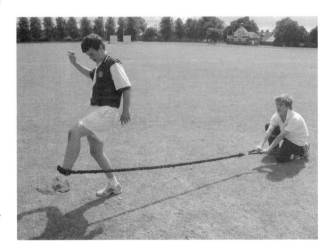

DRILL   PUNCH-KICK RESISTOR PARTNER DRILLS

Aim
To develop upper body strength and power.

Area/equipment
Indoor or outdoor area, 2 punch kick resistors per pair of youngsters.

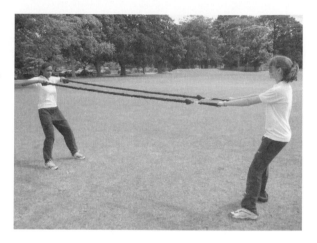

Description
Youngsters standing facing each other holding the punch kick resistors between them so they are flexed. The drill commences when one of the youngsters pulls the Flexi-cords towards their chest, similar to an upright rowing motion. On completing the row, partner now repeats the same drill. The drill is alternated from partner to partner until the required amounts of reps have been completed.

Key teaching points
- Stay tall
- Inhale on the effort (pull), exhale on the movement out
- Do not arch the back
- Do not sink into the hips
- Develop a rhythm.

Sets and reps
2 sets of 20 reps with 2 minutes recovery between each set.

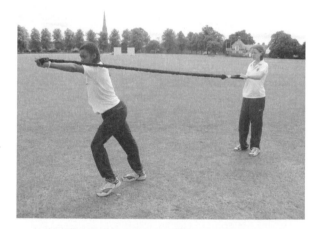

Variations/progressions
- Partner to hold punch kick resistor from behind so that forward punches can be performed.
- Partner to hold punch kick resistor in a seated position, so that arm curls or other types of resisted upper body drills can be performed.

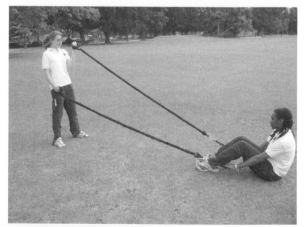

CHAPTER 6 EXPRESSION OF POTENTIAL

PRACTICAL APPLICATION OF ALL MOVEMENT SKILLS

This stage is short in duration, but very important. The youngsters will experience all the elements of the Youth Continuum in fun and even sometimes competitive situations. Short tag-type games and random agility tests work really well here. The key is to use all the movement skills that have been practised and improved through the Youth Continuum in real play situations. This stage also provides the opportunity to excite and challenge the youngsters. Most importantly, it will guarantee an exhilarating finish to a lesson, so as to ensure that the youngsters will be looking forward to the next one!

Because many of the possible activities can replicate the 'chaos' of games, this provides another excellent opportunity for the teacher/coach to evaluate how youngsters are moving once their attention is given to tactics and strategies at the same time.

Health and safety

■ Check movement directions and spacing

■ Create clearly marked playing areas.

DRILL CIRCLE BALL

Aim
To practise using explosive evasion skills.

Area/equipment
Outdoor or indoor area. Youngsters make a circle about 15 yards in diameter (depending on the size of the group). Foam balls/beanbags.

Description
One or two youngsters stand in the centre of the circle while the youngsters on the outside have 1 or 2 foam balls. The object is for those on the outside to try and make contact (with the ball) with those on the inside. The youngsters on the inside try to dodge the balls. The winners are the pair that has the fewest number of hits during their time in the centre.

Key teaching point
■ Youngsters on the inside should use the correct mechanics.

Sets and reps
Each pair to stay in the centre area for 45 seconds.

Variation/progression
■ Youngsters in the middle have to hold on to each other's hand or use a Break-Away Belt.

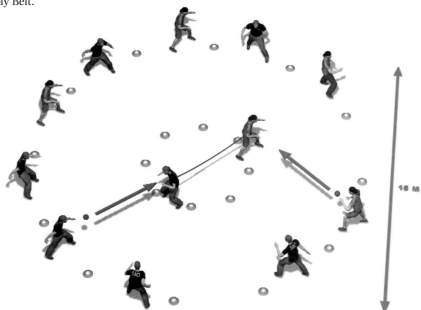

Figure 6.1 Circle ball

DRILL   ROBBING THE NEST

Aim
To practise multidirectional explosive speed, agility and quickness.

Area/equipment
Outdoor or indoor area of about 22 square yards, with a centre circle measuring 2 yards in diameter, marked out with markers. Place a number of foam balls/beanbags/tennis balls in the centre circle.

Description
Two nominated youngsters defend the 'nest' of the tennis balls with the rest of the youngsters standing on the outside of the square area. The game starts when the outside youngsters run in and try to steal the cricket balls from the nest and take them to the outside of the square, the 'safe zone'. The two defenders of the nest try to prevent the robbers from getting the cricket balls to the safe zone by tagging them or getting in their way. For every successful tag and prevention, the ball is returned to the centre circle.

Key teaching points
- Correct mechanics must be used at all times
- Youngsters should dodge, swerve, weave, sidestep, etc.
- Light contact only should be used
- Keep head up, use visual awareness at all times.

Sets and reps
Each pair to defend for about 45 seconds.

Variation/progression
- Attackers work in pairs, one attempts to retrieve the foam balls/beanbags/tennis balls from the middle by getting to the ball and rolling it out for the outer partner to field.

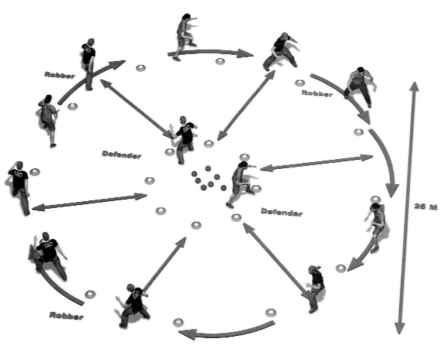

Figure 6.2 Robbing the nest

DRILL | ODD ONE OUT

Aim
To practise speed, agility and quickness in a competitive environment.

Area/equipment
Outdoor or indoor area; markers and cricket balls. Mark out a circle of 20–25 yards in diameter and a centre of about 2 yards in diameter.

Description
Place a number of foam balls/beanbags/tennis balls in the centre area, one fewer than the number of youngsters present. The youngsters are situated on the outside of the larger circle. On the teacher/coach's call the youngsters start running round the larger circle. On the teacher/coach's second call they collect a ball from the centre circle as quickly as possible. The youngster without a ball is the odd one out and performs an activity as directed by the teacher/coach while the next round is completed. The teacher/coach then removes another foam ball/beanbag/tennis ball and repeats the process.

Key teaching points
- Correct mechanics must be used at all times
- Youngsters should be aware of other youngsters around them.

Sets and reps
Play the game until a winner emerges.

Variation/progression
- Work in pairs joined together by holding hands or using the Break-Away Belt, one ball between 2 youngsters. If they break away from each other, they are disqualified.

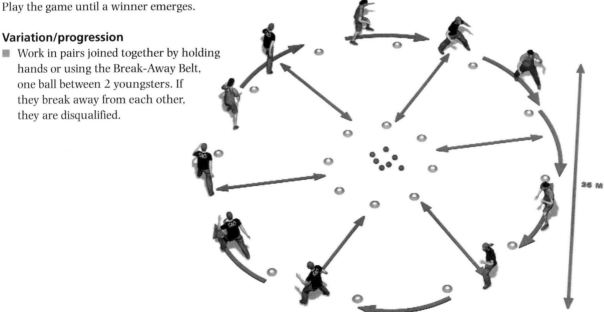

Figure 6.3 Odd one out

DRILL   *MARKER TURNS*

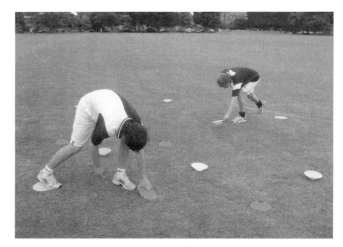

Aim
To practise multidirectional speed, agility and quickness.

Area/equipment
Outdoor or indoor area of about 20 square yards; 50 small markers. Place the markers in and around the grid; 25 of the markers should be turned upside down.

Description
Working in two small teams (2–3 youngsters), one team attempts to turn over the upright markers and the other team attempts to turn over the upside-down markers. The winners are the team that has the largest number of markers their way up after 60 seconds.

Key teaching points
■ Initiate good arm drive after turning a marker
■ Use correct multidirectional mechanics
■ Be aware of other youngsters around the area.

Sets and reps
A game should last for 60 seconds.

Variation/progression
■ Use 4 teams and allocate 4 different-coloured markers.

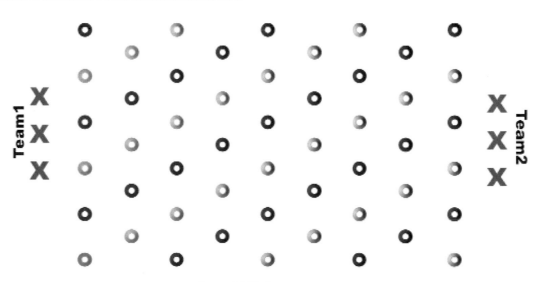

Figure 6.4 Marker turns

DRILL   TRUCKS AND TRAILERS

Aim
To practise multidirectional speed, agility and quickness reactions while mirroring another youngster's movements.

Area/equipment
Large outdoor or indoor area. Marker dots or cones.

Description
Working in pairs, one youngster leads (is the truck) while the other youngster follows just behind (is the trailer). The 'truck' moves in different directions and at different angles while the 'trailer' mirrors the exact movements. The roles are reversed after the recommended period of time.

Key teaching points
■ Initiate good arm drive after turning a marker
■ Use correct multidirectional mechanics
■ Be aware of other youngsters around the area
■ Keep a safe distance between the youngsters working together.

Sets and reps
A game should last for 60 seconds and then roles are to be reversed.

Variation/progression
■ Work in groups of 3 or 4.

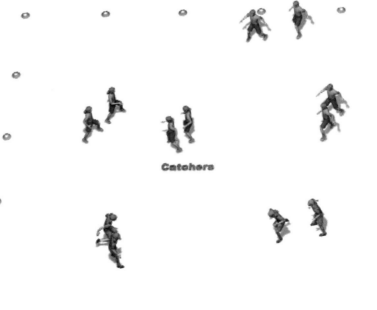

Figure 6.5 Trucks and trailers

DRILL | *SNAKE GAME*

Aim

To practise multidirectional speed, agility and quickness, co-ordination, balance and reactions while playing in a team environment.

Area/equipment

Use an indoor or outdoor area.

Description

The game starts off with 2 youngsters holding hands, while the other youngsters spread around the designated area. The object is for the first 2 youngsters to chase and tag other youngsters, without breaking hands. When tagged, the youngsters join hands with the chasers, therefore making a 'snake'. The game is finished when the final person is tagged.

Key teaching points

- Keep head up and be aware of others
- Use short steps when changing direction
- Youngsters who are being chased should use correct form of mechanics for movement.

Sets and reps

Play the game for 4–5 minutes depending on the size of the group.

Variation/progression

Have 2 snakes working together.

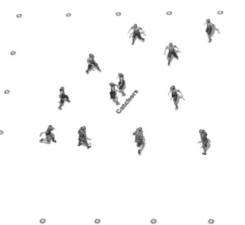

Figure 6.6(a) Snake game stage 1

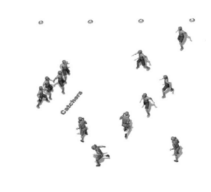

Figure 6.6(b) Snake game stage 2

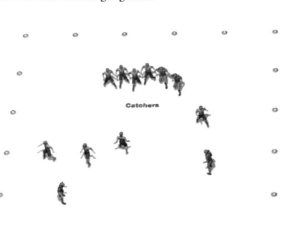

Figure 6.6(c) Snake game stage 3

DRILL | CONE GAME

Aim
To develop multidirectional patterns of movement; to utilise visual awareness in a team game.

Area/equipment
Use an indoor or outdoor grid using 4 coloured marker spots and 4 x 3 sets of cones the same colour as the marker spots. The 4 marker spots are placed in a 5-yard square. The 3 cones of the same colour are placed at a marker spot of a different colour.

Description
Four youngsters are placed one at each marker spot; the object of the game is for the youngster to move her or his 3 coloured cones to their corresponding coloured marker spot. The winner is the youngster who clears all the cones from her or his marker spot first.

Key teaching points
- Correct mechanics to be used at all times
- Youngsters should be encouraged to use sidesteps, dodges, swerves etc.
- Ensure youngsters keep heads up and are aware of the other youngsters.

Sets and reps
Play until the winner is decided.

Variation/progression
Increase marker spots and cones to 5–6 stations.

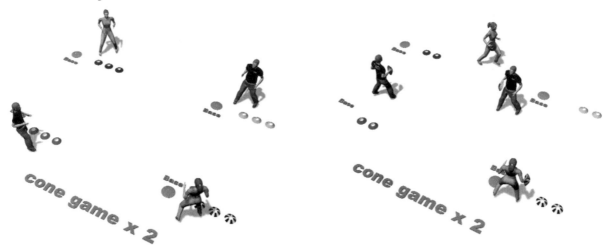

Figure 6.7(a) Cone game stage 1   Figure 6.7(b) Cone game stage 2

DRILL   *BRITISH BULLDOG*

Aim

To practise multidirectional explosive movements in a pressured situation.

Area/equipment

Outdoor or indoor area of approximately 20 square yards and about 20 markers to mark out start and finish lines.

Description

One youngster is nominated and stands in the centre of the grid, while the rest stand to one side. On the teacher/coach's call, all the youngsters attempt to get to the opposite side of the square without being caught by the youngster in the middle. When the youngster in the middle captures another youngster, she or he joins them in the middle and helps to capture more 'prisoners'.

Key teaching points

- Use correct mechanics at all times
- Keep head and eyes up to avoid collisions with other youngsters.

Sets and reps

Play British Bulldog for approximately 3–4 minutes before moving on to the more technical aspects of the game.

Variations/progressions

- The youngster in the middle uses a foam ball to touch other youngsters in order to capture them. The ball can be held or thrown
- Two youngsters linked by a Break-Away Belt stand in the middle and act as catchers. If the belt breaks apart while touching a runner the touch does not count,

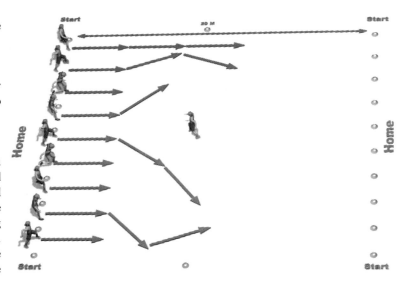

Figure 6.8(a) British bulldog

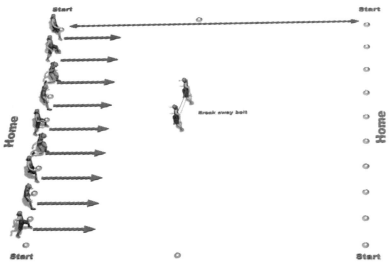

Figure 6.8(b) British bulldog using Break-Away Belt

CHAPTER 7 VISUAL AWARENESS

The usual 'eye test' experienced by most of us is concerned with Static Visual Acuity, i.e. the ability to identify a certain sized letter/number on an eye chart. This is not the only visual ability that a youngster needs to have in relation to sports performance. There are a number of categories that can be used to ascertain how a youngster uses vision in the performance of sports skills.

Static – Seeing static objects, e.g. sideline signals and scoreboards, clearly is desirable but not the most important thing.

Dynamic – Maintaining the clarity of an object in motion is vital to the timing of skills, and noticing depth and object variations.

Contrast – Discriminating the brightness and colour of an object against its background is key to the performance of batting skills, for example.

Colour – Spotting team-mates and following a moving object requires good colour recognition.

Eye movement - Shifting the eyes from place to place rapidly and accurately is essential to 'scanning' skills.

Accommodation – Rapidly changing focus will affect the clarity of objects as they move around in space.

Binocularity – Working the eyes together can affect all judgements of spatial orientation, e.g. following an incoming ball or person.

Depth perception – The need to judge distances and relationships to objects or places in space is vital in all activities.

Reaction Time – Making sense of and responding to stimuli quickly is increasingly important as the move towards elite performance is made.

Central/peripheral – Being aware of that which is to the sides, at the same time as looking at what is central, is a prerequisite for games players.

Eye–Hand–Body Co-ordination – Integrating the eyes and the hands/body as a unit is important at all levels of performance. Erratic and inconsistent movements will result if there are deficits in this ability.

Visual adjustability – Rapid adjustment to changing surroundings and environment at the same time as guiding the body's motor responses is necessary to meet the demands of playing in 'away' venues', for example.

Visualisation – Mentally rehearsing situations and actions can promote good performance and assist with the process of learning from mistakes.

Visual awareness can be developed within and at all stages of the SAQ Youth Continuum. Areas such as visual acuity, peripheral vision, tracking and depth perception can be included in many of the drills. This can add additional fun and challenges without the need to be too testing and scientific.

One simple method is to make use of the Visual Acuity Ring and the Peripheral Vision Stick.

DRILL   *VISUAL AWARENESS – FOLLOW THE THUMB*

Aim
To develop all-round and peripheral vision.

Area/equipment
Indoor or outdoor area, standing or seated.

Description
With either hand, hold arm out in front and make a 'thumbs up' sign. Keeping your head still and moving only your eyes, move the thumb up, down and around making sure you are moving to the extremes of your range of vision. Start slowly and increase the speed of the movement.

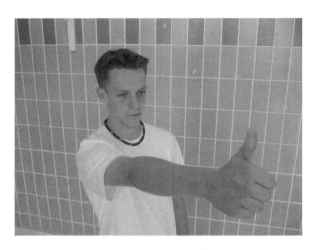

Key teaching points
- Sit upright with a good posture
- Try exercise with both left and right hands.

Sets and reps
Continue for 3 minutes in total.

Variation/progression
Practise drill in different lights, i.e. semi-dark to very bright.

DRILL VISUAL AWARENESS – VISUAL ACUITY RING

Aim
To develop visual acuity, tracking and manipulation skills in catching moving objects.

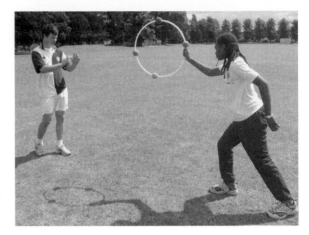

Area/equipment
Indoor or outdoor area and a visual acuity ring.

Description
Work in pairs approximately 5 yards apart; the ring is tossed between the youngsters so that it rotates through the air and is caught on the coloured ball nominated by the thrower or teacher/coach.
NB: don't spin ring too fast at the start as a youngster may shy away from it instead of catching it.

Key teaching points
■ Keep the head still
■ Move the eyes to track the ring
■ Work on the balls of the feet so that movement and adjustment can be made quickly
■ Hands should be held out in front of the body ready to catch the ring.

Sets and reps
2 sets of 10 reps with 1 minute recovery.

Variations/progressions
■ Increase the spin gradually
■ Vary the receiver's starting position, i.e. sideways, or facing away so he or she has to turn and catch
■ Receiver catches one- or two-handed
■ Ring is thrown horizontally
■ Youngster throws ring up and selects coloured ball to catch themselves
■ Spin the ring on the edge, i.e. like spinning a coin. Catch the selected ball before the ring hits the ground.

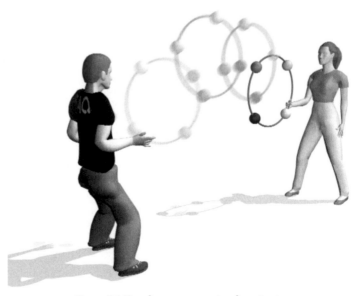

Figure 7.1 Visual awareness – visual acuity ring

DRILL   *VISUAL AWARENESS – NUMBERS AND LETTERS BALL*

Aim
To develop the ability to make subtle focus changes.

Area/equipment
Indoor or outdoor area, seated or standing and ball or beanbag.

Description
Draw numbers and letters all over the surface of a ball or beanbag. Toss it from hand to hand, back and forth, calling out as many numbers and letters as you can read each time.

Key teaching points
- Toss the ball/beanbag at steady pace
- Increase speed as you improve.

Sets and reps
Each set lasts for 1 minute. Do 3 sets with a 1 minute recovery between each set.

Variation/progression
Practise drill in different lights, i.e. semi-dark to very bright.

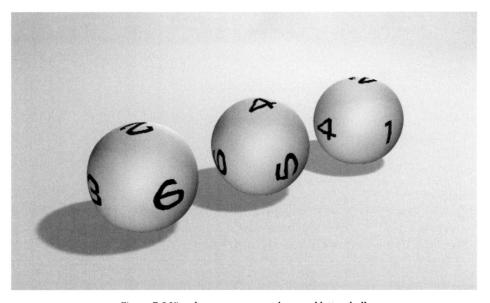

Figure 7.2 Visual awareness – numbers and letters ball

DRILL VISUAL AWARENESS – PERIPHERAL AWARENESS

Aim
To develop peripheral awareness; to help the youngster detect and react to the ball coming from behind and from the side more quickly.

Area/equipment
Outdoor or indoor area; use a Peripheral Vision Stick.

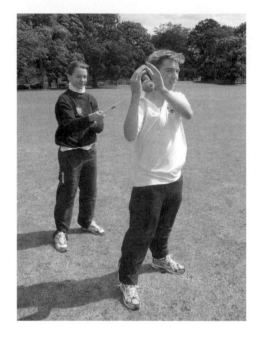

Description
Work in pairs with youngster 1 behind youngster 2 who stands in a ready position. Youngster 1 holds the stick and moves it from behind youngster 2 into his or her field of vision. As soon as youngster 2 detects the stick he or she claps both hands over the ball at the end of the stick.

Key teaching points
■ Youngster 2 should work off the balls of the feet and in a slightly crouched position with the hands held out ready
■ Youngster 1 must be careful not to touch any part of youngster 2's body with the stick
■ Youngster 1 should vary the speed at which the stick is brought into youngster 2's field of vision.

Sets and reps
2 set of 20 reps with no recovery between each rep and 1 minute recovery between each set.

Variations/progressions
■ Instead of using a vision stick, throw balls from behind youngster 2 that have to be fended off
■ A feeder at the back of youngster 2 pushes stick forward from side to side. Youngster 2 turns and claps ball
■ Youngster 2 claps ball fed from rear, turns to clap ball now fed from the front
■ Three feeders, one on either side, feeding in a ball to catch, alternated with one feeding in stick from behind to be clapped
■ Turn head to glance at ball fed from behind
■ Youngster 2 fends off stick, pushing it away with the outside of one hand
■ Repeat drills standing on one leg to enhance proprioception
■ Randomly receive stick end then ball end
■ Place a hand on shoulder before ball is lowered onto shoulder; hand moves to opposite shoulder
■ Increase speed of feeds by having 2 sticks and feeders.

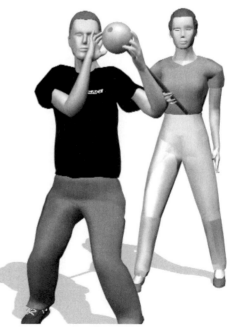

Figure 7.3 Visual awareness – peripheral awareness

DRILL VISION AND REACTION – BUNT BAT

Aim
To develop lightning-quick hand–eye co-ordination

Area/equipment
Outdoor or indoor area. Bunt Bat and tennis balls or beanbags.

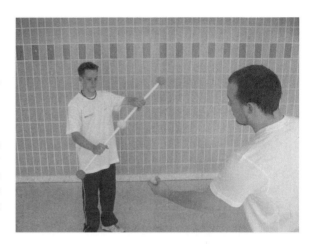

Description
Work in pairs; one of the youngsters holds the Bunt Bat. The partner stands about 3–4 yards away and throws a ball or beanbag, simultaneously calling the colour of one of the balls on the Bunt Bat. The youngster's task is to fend off the ball/beanbag with the appropriate coloured ball on the Bunt Bat.

Key teaching points
- Start throwing the balls/beanbag slowly and gradually build up the speed
- The youngster should be in a get-set position.

Sets and reps
3 sets of 25 reps with 30 seconds recovery between each set.

Variations/progressions
- Use different-coloured balls/beansbags – when the ball/beanbag has been thrown, it is to be fended off with the corresponding coloured ball on the Bunt Bat
- The youngster stands on an agility disc while performing the drill.

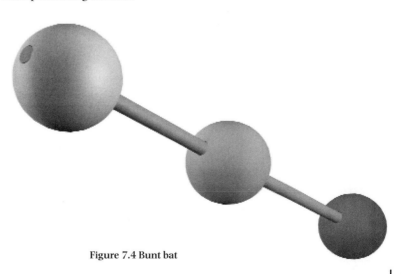

Figure 7.4 Bunt bat

CHAPTER 8 WARM DOWN, RECOVERY AND RELAXATION

After intense activity level, youngsters should be given time gradually to reduce the heart rate to near resting, and prepare for the next time that they are active again. Warming down and recovering properly will help to:

- Disperse lactic acid
- Prevent blood pooling
- Return the body systems to normal levels
- Assist in recovery.

The structure of the warm-down will be the Dynamic Flex warm-up movements and static stretches. It will last only a few minutes or more depending on the time available. The warm-down begins with moderate Dynamic Flex movements, which will gradually become less intense and smaller in amplitude. Throughout these exercises there should still be a focus on quality of movement and awareness of balance and general control of the body.

With the inclusion also of a series of static stretches, the warm-down is a time when the issue of flexibility can be explored and the youngsters are returned to a relaxed state.

Health and safety

- Encourage slow controlled movements
- Emphasise care when moving backwards.

DYNAMIC FLEX WARM-DOWN			
EXERCISE	INTENSITY	EXERCISE	INTENSITY
Butt kicks	50%	Walking hamstring	Walk
Hurdle walk	50%	Side lunge	Walk
Knee-out skip	40%	Quadriceps stretch	Static
Knee-across skip	40%	Hamstring stretch	Static
Low skips	30%	Adductors stretch	Static
Carioca	30%	Calf stretch	Static
Ankle flicks	20%	Gluteals stretch	Static

CHAPTER 9 USING SAQ IN SPORTS–SPECIFIC PRACTICES

This section provides examples of how to insert the SAQ principles and training drills into sports-specific practices. The primary aim is to improve the multidirectional explosive speed, agility, control, power and co-ordination required to perform quality sports movements. These drills also add additional challenges and variation to classes and sessions, thereby increasing the participant's motivation and enjoyment.

DRILL

RUNNING FORM –
STRIDE FREQUENCY AND STRIDE LENGTH

Aim

To practise the transfer from the acceleration phase to the increase in stride frequency and length required when running; to develop an efficient leg cycle, rhythm, power, foot placement, deceleration, control and balance when throwing and catching under pressure.

Area/Equipment

Indoor or outdoor area 40–60 yards long. Place 12 coloured stride frequency canes, marker dots or sticks at 3-, 4-, 5- and 6-foot intervals flat on the ground in a straight line. Sets of stumps/cones or small goals should be placed 60 cm after the last cane, and a marker dot or cone 60 cm from the front cane.

Description

Youngster 1 starts from behind the first cone. He or she steps round the cone and begins to accelerate down the stride frequency canes. The canes are laid out so that the initial stages for the run develop acceleration, therefore they are closer together; the middle part the canes are wider apart, which will develop stride length. The final few canes are closer again to develop deceleration. Youngster 1, on reaching the end canes, will now decelerate. As he or she is about to reach the set of stumps/cones or small goal at that end, youngster 2, who is standing behind them, throws or kicks the ball out at an angle along the ground; youngster 1 now reaccelerates to field the ball and returns it to youngster 2, who has now moved into a position to either hit the stumps with the ball, score a goal or touch the cone.

Sets and reps

1 set equals 6 reps with a walk-back recovery in between

Key teaching points

■ Do not overstride
■ Work off the balls of the feet
■ Try to develop and maintain a rhythm
■ Keep eyes and head up as if looking over a fence
■ Maintain correct mechanics
■ Maintain an upright posture
■ Stay focused.

Variations/progressions

■ Varied starting positions
■ Run in pairs.

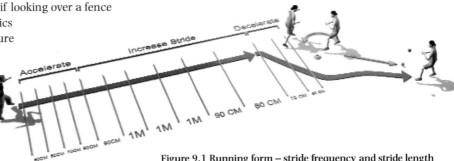

Figure 9.1 Running form – stride frequency and stride length

DRILL

RUNNING FORM – STRIDE FREQUENCY AND STRIDE LENGTH ADVANCED FIELDING

Aim

To practise the transfer from the acceleration phase to the increase in stride frequency and length required when running; to develop an efficient leg cycle, rhythm, power, foot placement, deceleration, control and balance when throwing and catching under pressure in a more complex and advanced situation.

Area/equipment

Indoor or outdoor area 40–60 yards long. Place 2 lines of 12 coloured stride frequency canes, marker dots or sticks at 3-, 4-, 5- and 6-foot intervals flat on the ground in a straight line, 10 yards apart. A set of stumps should be placed in the middle between the 2 lines of stride frequency canes. Marker dots should be placed at the beginning of each line of canes.

Description

Two youngsters, 1 and 2, simultaneously commence their run down the stride frequency canes A and B. On nearing the end, coach X, standing 15–20 yards away between both lines of canes, throws the ball along the ground at an angle away from youngster 1. Youngster 1 now runs to field the ball; youngster 2 turns and accelerates to the stumps situated between the sets of canes. Youngster 1, on fielding the ball, throws the ball over the stumps to youngster 2, who touches the stumps then returns the ball to coach X. The drill is then repeated on the other side.

Key teaching points

- Do not overstride
- Work off the balls of the feet
- Try to develop and maintain a rhythm
- Keep eyes and head up as if looking over a fence
- Maintain correct mechanics
- Maintain an upright posture
- Stay focused
- Alter distances between strides for different ages and heights.

Sets and reps

1 set of 4 reps.

Variations/progressions

- Runners to work through the grid with ball in hand
- The drill can be made continuous by starting from both ends.

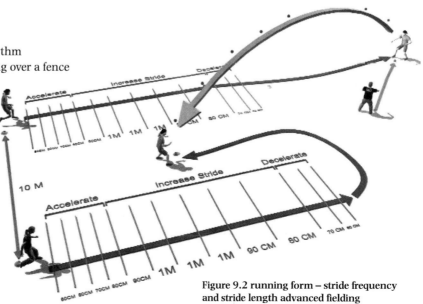

Figure 9.2 running form – stride frequency and stride length advanced fielding

DRILL

INTEGRATING RUNNING
FORM WITH GAME SKILL DEVELOPMENT

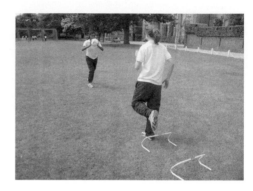

Aim

To develop correct, precise and controlled lateral stepping movements while manipulating or striking a ball.

Area/equipment

Indoor or outdoor area. Place 3 hurdles side by side about 18 inches apart.

Description

Youngster stands on the outside of either hurdle 1 or hurdle 3 so that he or she will step over the middle of each hurdle. The youngster performs lateral movement mechanics while clearing each hurdle; on clearing hurdle 3, he or she repeats the drill in the opposite direction. A ball/beanbag or frisbee can now be introduced.

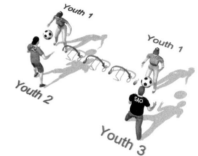

Figure 9.3(a) Groups of 3

Key teaching points

- Maintain correct lateral running form/mechanics
- Maintain correct arm mechanics
- Do not sink into the hips
- Keep the head up
- Do not lean too far forwards
- Use small steps and work off the balls of the feet
- Do not use an excessively high knee-lift.

Sets and reps

2 sets of 6 reps, 3 to the left and 3 to the right, with a 60 second recovery between sets.

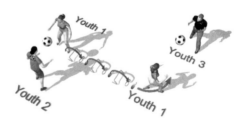

Figure 9.3(b) With a turn

Variations/progressions

- Work with a teacher/coach, who should randomly direct the youngster over the hurdles
- Add 2 Macro V Hurdles to add lift variations
- Work in groups of 3: youngster 1 works through the hurdles; youngster 2 and youngster 3 stand at either end and throw the ball for youngster 1 to catch as he or she gets to their end (see fig 9.3(a)
- Youngster 1 can also turn after they have stepped over the last hurdle and receive the ball from another youngster (see fig 9.3(b)
- Use 6 hurdles. Youngster 1 performs mechanic drill down the hurdles. Coach stands 2 yards away from the last hurdle at a set of stumps or cone. Youngster 1 comes over the last hurdle, coach throws or kicks ball to the left or right of the hurdles for the youngster to accelerate to and return to the coach (see fig 9.3(c)).

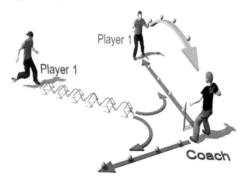

Figure 9.3(c) Accelerating onto ball

DRILL   RUNNING FORM – FIELDING DRILL

Aim

To develop and maintain a high level of running performance while under pressure in the field to catch, kick or receive a ball.

Area/equipment

Outdoor or indoor, large area of 40–60 yards. Place out a line of 16 hurdles: the first 8 hurdles should be 2 feet apart, then a 5-yard gap, then the next line of 8 hurdles continues at 2 feet apart. Marker A is placed at the start, 1 yard away from the first hurdle; marker B is placed between the 8th and 9th hurdles. Football, cricket ball, tennis ball, netball, basketball etc.

Description

From marker A youngster1 performs a drill down the first set of hurdles. Youngster 2 (with ball in hand) waits at marker B for youngster 1 to reach the centre gap. As youngster 1 clears the final hurdle, youngster 2 throws the ball out at an angle to the left or right of the centre gap, then immediately turns and commences a drill down the second set of hurdles towards the stumps. On clearing the final hurdle, youngster 2 now accelerates behind the stump. Youngster 1, who has accelerated off to field the ball, now throws it back to youngster 2.

Key teaching points

- Maintain correct arm mechanics
- Work off the balls of the feet
- Try to develop and maintain a rhythm
- Keep eyes and head up and look ahead
- Maintain an upright posture
- Keep the hips square.

Sets and reps

4 sets of 4 reps.

Variations/progressions

- Perform the drills laterally
- Youngster 2 to kick/throw
  2 balls for youngster 1 to retrieve

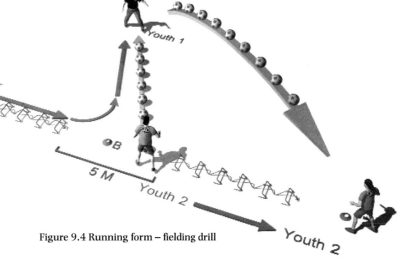

Figure 9.4 Running form – fielding drill

DRILL GAME-SPECIFIC HURDLE MIRROR DRILLS

Aim
To improve the performance of mechanics under pressure. To improve random agility, balance and co-ordination.

Area/equipment
Indoor or outdoor area. Mark out a grid with 2 lines of 8 hurdles, with 2 feet between each hurdle and 2 yards between each line of hurdles.

Description
First-to-the-ball drill: youngsters face each other while performing drills up and down the lines of hurdles. A ball is placed between the 2 lines of hurdles. The proactive youngster commences the drill as normal then accelerates to the ball, fields it and sprints past the end cones. The reactive youngster attempts to beat the proactive youngster to the ball.

Key teaching points
- Stay focused on your partner
- The reactive youngster should try to anticipate the proactive youngster's movements
- Maintain correct arm mechanics
- Ensure correct technical skills are used when kicking or catching the ball.

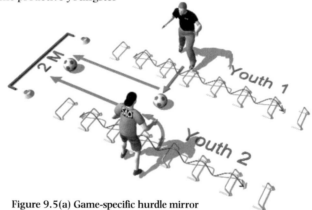

Figure 9.5(a) Game-specific hurdle mirror drills – using ball

Sets and reps
Each youngster performs 3 sets of 30-second work periods. Ensure 30 seconds recovery between each work period.

Variations/progressions
- Vary the movement drills down the hurdles
- Mirror drill can be performed using racquets, hockey sticks etc. to simulate movements used in the game

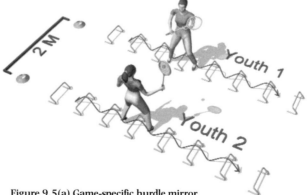

Figure 9.5(a) Game-specific hurdle mirror drills – using racquets

DRILL
INTEGRATING RUNNING
FORM WITH LATERAL GAMES SKILLS

Aim
To develop efficient and economical lateral sidesteps while catching and throwing the ball.

Area/equipment
Indoor or outdoor area. Place 8 Micro V Hurdles side on, 1 yard apart and staggered laterally. Position a finish marker in the same pattern as the hurdles.

Description
Youngster 1 works inside the channel created by the hurdles and steps over each hurdle with one foot as he or she moves laterally down and across the channel. On stepping over the outside hurdle a ball is thrown to him or her to catch and return by youngster 2 situated on one side. This action is also repeated on the opposite side with youngster 3. After receiving the ball youngsters 2 and 3 walk backwards into position ready for the next time youngster 1 steps over the outside hurdle.

Key teaching points
- Bring the knee up 45 degrees over the hurdle
- Do not overstride across the hurdle
- Maintain correct arm mechanics/strong arm drive
- Keep the hips square
- Do not sink into the hips.

Sets and reps
2 sets of 3 reps with a walk-back recovery between reps and 2 minutes between sets.

Variation/progression
Perform the drill backwards.

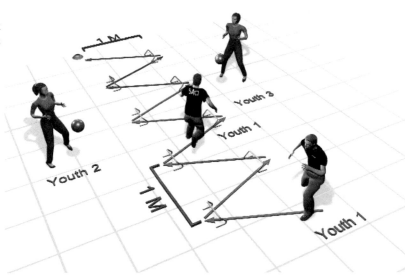

FAST FOOT LADDER –
WITH FIELDING, THROWING AND KICKING

Aim
To develop fast feet, balance, co-ordination and agility while fielding a ball in the outfield.

Area/equipment
Large indoor or outdoor area. Ladders, stumps, small goal or cone, foam/tennis/cricket ball etc. Place 3 sets of ladder sections next to each other, 2 yards apart at one end. The central ladder (ladder A) will be straight; the ladders on each side (B and C) will be angled away so that they are both 4 yards away from ladder A at the other end. 10 yards on from the end of ladder A is a set of stumps or small goal or cone.

Description
Youngster 1 starts on ladder A, youngsters 2 and 3 start on ladders B and C respectively. On the coaches call, all three commence fast foot drills down his or her ladder. As they get near to the end of the ladders, the coach, who is situated beyond the stumps, will throw, roll or kick a ball out to the left of ladder C. Youngster 1 accelerates from ladder A to cover the stumps/goal/cone, youngster 2 accelerates from ladder B behind youngster 1 to back up the kick/throw, youngster 3 accelerates out of ladder C to the ball and return it to youngster 1 over the stumps/goal/cone. Youngster 1 can either hit the stumps, score a goal or touch the cone with the ball. Youngsters are now rotated to different starting positions.

Key teaching points
- Maintain correct running form/mechanics
- Ensure that correct technical skills are used when youngsters are throwing, kicking and catching the ball.
- Youngsters should communicate clearly – both visually and verbally.

Sets and reps
3 sets of 6 reps with 1 minute recovery between each set, i.e. 3 reps as youngsters 1, 3 reps as youngster 2 and 3 reps as youngster 3.

Variation/progression
Vary the fast foot ladder drills performed linearly and laterally by the youngsters.

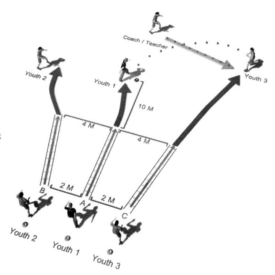

DRILL

FAST FOOT LADDER –
LATERAL THROWING AND CATCHING

Aim
To develop fast foot combination work, balance, co-ordination, acceleration, timing and throwing and catching laterally under pressure.

Area/equipment
Large indoor or outdoor area. Place 3 sections of 15 foot ladder 5 yards apart and 1 stump 10 yards away at the end of each ladder as shown below in fig. x.x. Use cricket ball, tennis ball, baseball, softball, etc.

Description
Youngster 1 accelerates down ladder A; youngsters 2 and 3 also accelerate down their corresponding ladders B and C. As youngster 1 leaves ladder A, coach X will throw a ball for him or her to catch and then throw on to youngster 2, who then throws the ball to youngster 3, who catches and throws the ball on to coach Y. On completion of their throws, the youngsters accelerate to the end stumps A, B and C; coach Y now nominates one of the youngsters and throws him or her the ball to catch and knock the stump. The youngsters now jog back to the start and the drill is then repeated from the opposite side.

Key teaching points
■ Maintain correct running form/mechanics
■ Youngsters should communicate
■ Good timing of support runs is important
■ Good throwing and catching techniques are to be used.

Sets and reps
3 sets of 5 reps with a slow jog back recovery between reps and a 2 minute recovery between each set.

Variations/progressions
■ Vary the ladder drills
■ Vary the type of throw
■ Ball can be rolled to be fielded
■ Vary the youngsters' starting positions between the 3 ladders
■ Use a football; youngsters kick the ball instead of throwing it

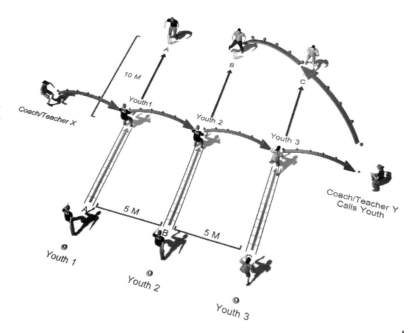

DRILL

FAST FOOT LADDER –
FIELDING GIANT CROSSOVER

Aim
To develop fast feet, speed, agility, co-ordination, visual, reaction and fielding skills both with and without the ball.

Area/equipment
Large indoor or outdoor area. Place 4 ladders in a cross formation with 25 yards between them in the centre area; 2 or 4 foam/tennis balls, footballs, netballs, basketballs, etc.

Description
Split the youngsters into 4 equal groups and locate them at the start of each ladder A, B, C and D. Simultaneously, youngsters accelerate down the ladder performing fast foot drills. On coming out of the ladder in the centre area the 2 youngsters with a ball will either pick it up or dribble it across the centre and pass it to the oncoming youngster, who fields the ball before repeating the same action to the next oncoming youngster. Having fielded the ball, the youngster now joins the queue at the ladder on the opposite side of the cross without travelling down it.

Key teaching points
- This should be a continuous drill
- Maintain correct running form/mechanics
- Correct technical skills must be used when youngsters are on the ball
- Youngsters should use clear communication.

Sets and reps
3 sets of 6 reps with 1 minute recovery between each set.

Variations/progressions
- Instead of rolling the ball introduce throw and catch
- Hitting and striking of a ball can also be introduced here. This is highly skilled

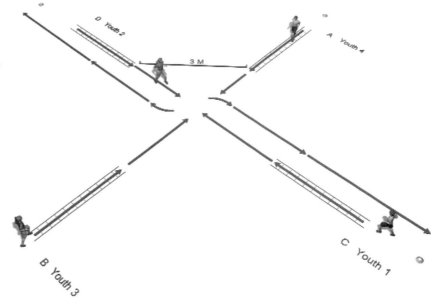

FAST FOOT LADDER –

DRILL   **FIELDING, BACKUP AND THROW**

Aim
To develop acceleration, balance and control while chasing a
foam/tennis/cricket ball in the deep outfield. Practise back-up
running, throwing and catching.

Area/equipment
Large indoor or outdoor area, 3 ladders, 2 markers and foam/tennis
balls. Stagger 2 ladders, A and B, 2 yards apart, 1 in front of the other.
5 yards in front of the starting ladder a third ladder C is laid laterally
(see diagram). Marker X is placed 20 yards away but directly in line
with ladder A, a second marker Y is placed 10 yards away laterally
across from ladder C.

Description
Youngster 1 starts his or her run down ladder A and accelerates out of
the ladder towards marker X. Coach standing near marker X rolls the
balls towards it, for youngster 1 to field. Youngster 2 times his or her
run to start after youngster 1 has passed him or her on the inside,
accelerates down ladder B to back up youngster 1. On reaching the ball
youngster 1 flicks it up to youngster 2, who catches it and throws
towards marker Y. Youngster 3, timing his or her run, accelerates
down lateral ladder C, arrives at marker Y in time to catch the ball and
throw it back to the coach standing on marker X.

Key teaching points
- Maintain good arm mechanics
- Keep head and eyes up
- Use correct throwing and
  catching technique.

Sets and reps
3 sets of 6 reps with 1 minute
recovery between each rep.

Variation/Progression
Vary ladder drills.

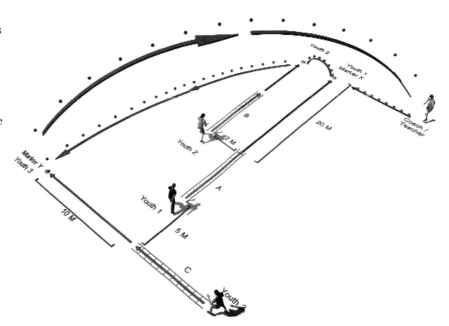

DRILL

CATCHING / STRIKING
LATERAL POWER AND SPEED DEVELOPMENT

Aim
To develop explosive, controlled lateral ability, and precise and acurate catching/striking of the ball at speed under pressure.

Area/equipment
Indoor or outdoor area, Viper Belt with 2 flexicords (1 attached at each side), cone, 2 x 7.5 feet fast feet ladder and ball (tennis, cricket, football, netball, etc).

Description
Youngster 1 is connected to youngsters 2 and 3 by the Viper Belt and 2 flexi-cords. The ladders are placed 1–2 yards behind the cone laterally on each side, leaving a gap for youngster 1 to stand in. Youngster 1 stands behind the cone, in-between the 2 ladders, while youngsters 2 and 3 provide resistance from both sides. Youngster 4 stands in front of the centre gap and throws or bounces balls each side of the centre cone, youngster 1 moves laterally down the ladders under resistance from one side and catches or returns the ball by hitting it with a racquet/bat. The drill is now repeated on the other side for the required number of reps. The Viper Belt is removed and the drill is performed without resistance (contrast phase).

Key teaching points
- Re-assert good arm mechanics when possible
- Maintain correct running form
- Use correct techniques for catching and throwing.

Sets and reps
3 sets of 8 reps plus 2 contrast, with 3 minutes recovery between each set.

Variations/progressions
- Can be performed without the ladders
- Work in sand pit or use high jump landing mats so that youngster 1 can dive for the ball
- Youngsters to wear appropriate kit, i.e. wicket keeper's gloves, goal keeper's gloves, etc

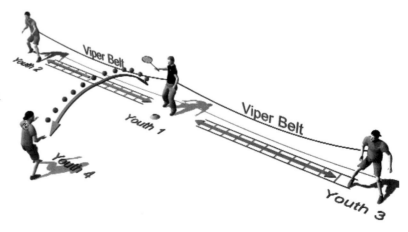

POSITION SPECIFIC –

DRILL | **BOWLER - ASSISTED RESISTED TOW RUNS**

Aim
To develop explosive run-up and power for bowling.

Area/equipment
Indoor or outdoor area, Viper Belt, wicket and cricket ball.

Description
Bowler 1 and 2 are attached to one another by the Viper Belt. Bowler 1 runs away from bowler 2, who stands still until pulled forward. Bowler 1 has the ball in his or her hand and attempts to run and bowl in normal fashion, while being resisted behind from bowler 2.

Key teaching points
- Maintain correct running form and mechanics
- Both bowlers should use strong arm drive
- Both bowlers should use short steps during the acceleration phase.
- Bowler 2 (the assisted bowler) must keep an upward and forward lean and not try to resist the acceleration by leaning back.

Sets and reps
2 sets of 6 reps; bowler to take 30 seconds recovery between each set and 2 minutes recovery between each rep.

Variation/progression
Bowler 2 to run with hand
    weights.

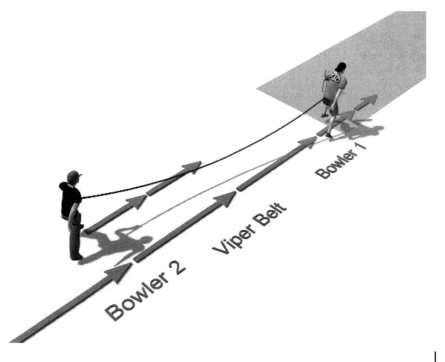

DEVELOPING SKILFUL MOVEMENT

As previously stated there is tremendous flexibility in how this programme can be used to improve all elements of youngsters' movement.

It will be helpful when structuring units of work for the school situation or training programmes for sports performers to consider how youngsters learn most easily. Skill learning is best taught progressing from simple to complex skills, and from general to specific skills, e.g. perform a good Dead Leg movement (see page 55) before attempting the more complicated Icky Shuffle (page 82) and establish good movement mechanics in the ladders before including a throw-and-catch routine.

Allow youngsters to learn by first seeing a clear demonstration of the activity and being given simple instructions on what they should do. If they are able to explore the new skills, they discover what they can already do and then experiment with the new movement challenges, for example, it may be that moving sideways along a ladder is performed adequately with feet going into the spaces, but the youngster's hips are twisted. The new focus is to try and keep the hips parallel with the black band of the ladder.

This movement can then be combined with, for example, catching a ball at the end of the ladder. The activity can be put into context by application to a 3 v. 1 game situation where, perhaps, the youngster moves sideways behind the defender to find a space to receive a pass. This puts the performer in a situation where he or she learns to select appropriate movements and apply them to the game. With sufficient practice, lateral movement using effective push off the trailing foot and quick, lateral steps with fast arms are consolidated and refined. Adaptation and extension of the movement vocabulary takes place when the youngster then decides to dodge sideways the 'other way' with a 'feint', before losing the defender to receive a pass with added time and space. (See *QCA Schemes of Work for Physical Education*).

Another example of this process is given in the Appendix, page 170.

Once a range of skills has been selected and practised by youngsters moving through the process just outlined, it may be useful for the teacher/coach to reflect on the performance by considering the 'Building Bricks Guide' below. This will allow movements to be made easier or harder depending on the level of success achieved by the performers.

'Building bricks' guide

Activities and practices can be modified using the following practice framwork. This is particularly useful during the exploratory phase of learning and to challenge pupils further once a skill has been mastered.

Quality (What you want to see in every movement!)

HOW			WHERE	
SPEED	**EFFICIENCY**	**DIRECTION**	**LEVEL**	**POSITION**
fast	light	on the spot	tall	own space
slow	heavy	forwards	short	on
go faster (accelerate)	Smooth	backwards	high	over
go slower (decelerate)	jerky	sideways	low	under
slow motion	softly	left/right	up	behind
fast/slow erratic	noisily	diagonal	down	in front
sustained	with spring	zigzag		between
stopping	with rhythm	straight line		around
	with/without arms	curve		beside
	explode	pattern		in and out
		twist		together
		turn		at the same time

Adapted from David L. Gallahue, *Movement Concepts*.

Planning a programme

To organise the inclusion of SAQ Training into a scheme of work or a year's sports training programme, several approaches may be considered: integration into existing sessions, following the SAQ Continuum, and creating SAQ sessions and building SAQ activities around the development of fundamental manipulation skills are just some possibilities.

Because SAQ Training may be seen as a tool to enhance teaching and coaching that is already in place, it is easy to integrate into an existing programme using the following guidelines and the sample lesson plans shown in the Appendix (page 170). NB: Teaching/Coaching points will also be found in previous pages.

Regardless of which of the suggested approaches is used, it may be worthwhile to consider beginning youngster's SAQ work with an introductory session. It is important that youngsters are helped to understand why they are doing SAQ activities and how and where these movements will contribute to their athletic progress. The aim would be to get youngsters to explore what contributes to 'Good Movement':

Q: – Why does one youngster appear to move more quickly than another?
A: – Because she runs on 'light' feet.
Q: – What makes the feet go faster?
A: – Fast arms.

This can be done by playing simple tag games. Another option, in athletics for example, would be to have youngsters observe their peers in short races. Why is Brian the fastest? Sarah does not win but looks a better runner, why? Once some of the questions have been discussed, youngsters can be introduced to improving their movement by using Mechanics.

Now that an understanding of the SAQ activities featured above has been achieved it should be possible to ensure that appropriate drills are put in place regardless of the ability of the performer. Differentiation can be achieved by focusing on the simple drills and changing the equipment, space, distances, time taken to perform, and number of repetitions, and reducing the number and type of movements in a sequence.

INTRODUCTORY LESSON	
AREA OF ACTIVITY	**Games or Athletics Activity: Fundamental movement**
TOPIC	Introduction to running
KEY STAGE 3	
LESSON AIM	To develop understanding of what is involved in 'good athletic movement'.
LESSON OBJECTIVE	To introduce youngsters to correct running actions.
Warm-up	Dynamic Flex (5 mins) 2 lines of youngsters moving forwards and backwards Jogs, skips, lateral lunges, hamstring walks, selection of short sprints.
Game	British Bulldog (5 mins) Key questions: ■ What is the best part of the foot to run on? ■ What is the best way of using the arms? ■ If the arms go fast what happens to the feet? ■ Is it best to take small or large steps? ■ Why is good balance important? ■ What role does the head play in movement?
Mechanics	To move on the balls of the feet.
Hurdles	(5 mins) – lines of 3 hurdles: Dead Leg, Leading Leg Run, Stride.
Game	(5 mins) Repeat British Bulldog with the focus being on how the feet are working. Indoors, ask youngsters to 'listen' to their feet. Quick light movement = no noise!
Mechanics	(5 mins) – Introduce correct arm action and repeat the above drills.
Game	(5 mins) Repeat the game with the focus on improved and faster arm action. To maintain interest change the rules.
Warm-down	(5 mins) – Slow Dynamic Flex movements repeated, plus static stretches.

Integration into existing sessions

An integrated approach allows existing schemes of work or training programmes to be modified simply with all skill development being underpinned by SAQ foundations.

8–LESSON DEVELOPMENT

1. Dynamic Flex, Mechanics, Skills, Game (Expression), Warm-down (WD)

2. Dynamic Flex, Mechanics, Skills, Game, WD

3. Dynamic Flex, Fast Feet, Skills, Game, WD

4. Dynamic Flex, Fast Feet, Skills, Game, WD

5. Dynamic Flex, Fast Feet, Skills, Game, WD

6. Dynamic Flex, Accumulation, Skills, Explosion, Game, WD

7. Dynamic Flex, Explosion, Skills, Game, WD

8. Dynamic Flex, Explosion, Skills, Game, WD

This can be illustrated using fig. 11.1

APPLICATION IN A UNIT OF WORK

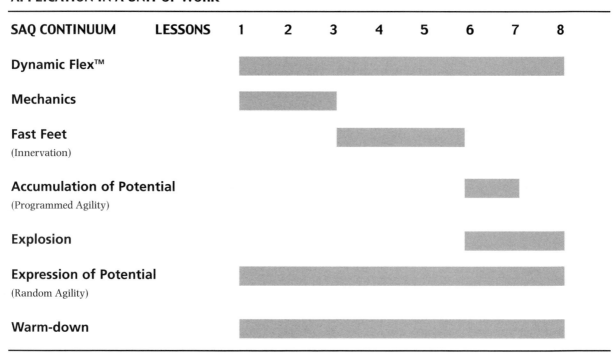

Figure 11.1 SAQ SCHOOLS PROGRAMME

SAMPLE INTEGRATION LESSON PLAN: Lesson 6	
AREA OF ACTIVITY	**Games: Multidirectional Movement Development**
TOPIC	Introduction to Programmed Agility and Explosive Starts
KEY STAGE 3	
LESSON AIM	To develop the ability to change direction with speed and precision; to evaluate the progress of youngsters.
LESSON OBJECTIVE	To improve patterns of movement and acceleration.
Warm-up	Dynamic Flex (5 mins) 2 lines of youngsters moving forwards and backwards; perform jogs, skips, lateral lunges, hamstring walks, selection of short sprints including Get-Ups.
Accumulation	(15 mins) Set up Team Circuit (see page 105). Allow youngsters to 'have a go'. Encourage them to observe performance, particularly when the speed of each run is increased (if appropriate, set up some races). NB: good mechanics will quickly disappear!
Skills	(10 mins) e.g. shooting a ball. NB: To have a chance to shoot, the youngster must have successfully outwitted an opponent to continue with the dribble or find space so as to receive the pass. This requires multidirectional movement patterns. Practice – youngsters move forwards, sideways and in zigzags before making a shot.
Explosion	(5 mins) In pairs, introduce Let Goes. NB: This can be introduced separately during the next lesson if lesson time is restricted.
Expression	(Game – 10 mins) Encourage elusive running and explosive acceleration through gaps.
Warm-down	(5 mins) Slow Dynamic Flex movements repeated and static stretches.

FOLLOWING SAQ CONTINUUM LESSONS

The SAQ Continuum can be used in its entirety to provide the structure to session planning where the focus is on developing sound movement principles as a foundation to activity-specific work to follow. This allows good movement to be constantly emphasised in all subsequent work. It can be used to lay down all the basic movement principles at the start of a year or the beginning of a key stage, and has been successfully used in Sports Colleges as part of a Transition Curriculum (Y6–Y7).

6–LESSON DEVELOPMENT

Lesson Theme: LINEAR movement

1. **LINEAR movement** Dynamic Flex, GAME (context), Mechanics, Game, Warm-down (WD).

2. **LINEAR movement** Dynamic Flex, Mechanics, Fast Feet, Game, WD.

3. **LINEAR movement** Dynamic Flex, Mechanics, Fast Feet, Game, WD.

4. **LATERAL movement** Dynamic Flex, Mechanics, Fast Feet, Game, WD.

5. **DECELERATE, ACCELERATE, PROGRAMMED AGILITY** Dynamic Flex, Accumulation of Potential Circuit, Game, WD.

6. **EXPLOSION** Dynamic Flex, Fast Feet, Explosion, Game, WD.

Such a format was also used in the successful research project conducted by Leeds Metropolitan University (Bailey and Morley)

SAMPLE CONTINUUM LESSON PLAN: Lesson 4	
AREA OF ACTIVITY	**Games: Multidirectional Movement Development**
TOPIC	Introduction to Lateral Movement
KEY STAGE 3	
LESSON AIM	To develop the ability to move sideways with balance and control; to improve the ability to dodge in a simple game.
LESSON OBJECTIVE	To improve patterns of movement and acceleration.
Warm-up	Dynamic Flex (5 mins) Youngsters moving forwards and backwards and sideways from own marker spot performing basic movements.
Mechanics	(10 mins) ■ Introductory activity – practise sidestepping, pushing off between 2 spots or between 2 lines. ■ 2 hurdles lateral step. Progress to 3 hurdles.
Innervation (Fast Feet)	(10 mins) Short ladders – lateral steps, repeat in and out, lateral Dead-Leg, mirror work
Expression	(Game – 10 mins) Circle Ball
Warm-down	(5 mins) Slow Dynamic Flex movements repeated plus static stretches.

MANIPULATION SKILL DEVELOPMENT USING SAQ

Another possible approach with the aim of providing a focus on the development of a wide range of fundamental movement skills is to use the SAQ Continuum in the following way:

1. **Throw – Catch**
   Dynamic Flex, SKILLS + Mechanics, Game, WD.

2. **Throw – Catch**
   Dynamic Flex, SKILLS + Mechanics, Game, WD.

3. **Passing – Feet**
   Dynamic Flex, SKILLS, Fast Feet, Game, WD.

4. **Dribbling – Bounce**
   Dynamic Flex, SKILLS, Fast Feet, Game, WD.

5. **Shooting – Hand**
   Dynamic Flex, Short Circuits to develop positioning for shooting, Game, WD.

6. **Shooting – Feet**
   Dynamic Flex, Short Circuits to develop positioning for shooting, Game, WD.

SAMPLE MANIPULATION SKILL DEVELOPMENT LESSON PLAN: Lesson 4	
AREA OF ACTIVITY	**Games: Develop Co-ordination**
TOPIC	Dribbling – Feet
KEY STAGE 3. YEAR 9	
LESSON AIM	To develop the ability to control a ball at the feet while moving.
LESSON OBJECTIVE	To develop the co-ordination necessary to dribble a ball while stationary and while moving at speed
Warm-up	Dynamic Flex (10 mins) Split Grid using footballs.
Skills	(5 mins) Free practice of dribbling ball around a grid in relation to another youngster and putting down cones to provide obstacles. Time challenge to finish, e.g. how many corners and cones dribbled around in 30 seconds.
Innervation (Fast Feet)	(10 mins) ■ Long Ladders – linear Dead-Leg, Leading-Leg Run, Icky Shuffle, practise repeat stepping out to touch, with foot, marker spots placed at sides of ladder; step back into ladder before moving forwards. Icky Shuffle practice ■ Add ball – Move through short ladder, collect ball and try to use similar small steps and good footwork at the same time as dribbling the ball across a grid. Short ladder crossovers dribbling ball across grid.
Expression (Game)	(10 mins) ■ Small-sided game with rules conditioned to promote dribbling, e.g. no passing in last third of pitch and restricted shooting area. ■ Rob The Nest to finish (optional).
Warm-down	(5 mins) Slow Dynamic Flex movements repeated and static stretches.

Good practice

What follows is an example of 'Good Practice' from an innovative sports college: Sedgefield Community College in Sedgefield, County Durham. This scheme of work for Year 7 (11–12-year olds) illustrates the way in which the SAQ Continuum has been successfully integrated into the first of a series of six games lessons.

YEAR 7 BOYS – SKILLS

(written by Steven Hepples, PE Dept, Sedgefield Community College (Sports College)

Area of Activity: GAMES	**Activity**: Movement skills		**Topic**: Introduction (tag games)
Key stage: 3	**Year**: 7	**Lesson No**: 1	**NC Level**: 3,4,5

Lesson Aim: To introduce pupils to equipment and key terminology to be used throughout the unit

Learning Objectives
- Pupils to perform all basic circuit incorporating all basic movement skills
- Pupils identify associated skills with specific sporting situations

	Resources

Starter Activity
■ Brainstorm – group discussion – Why do we need to move efficiently when playing sport?
■ Teacher-led warm-up – directed tasks focusing on varied movement in game situations
Main Learning
■ SAQ movement circuit (demonstration and completion). Pupils complete 8 different stations
   ■ Form and mechanics – core stability and co-ordination drills (e.g. hopping over hurdles)
   ■ Reactions – reflex reactions (e.g. stimulus response catch, reaction ball)
   ■ Fast feet – running speed and quickness (e.g. fast feet ladder drills)
   ■ Agility – stability and change of direction (e.g. Illinois course, marking drill activities)
■ At each station pupils are to answer the questions (on whiteboards): What sports? What skill?
■ Game – pupils have a game of tag rugby (running in any direction) – identify movement skills
Plenary
■ Teacher-led cool-down – dynamic flex
■ Group discussion and review of learning objectives (key questions)
■ Why do we need to move efficiently? What sports require require specific movement skills?
	■ SAQ ladders
	■ SAQ hurdles
	■ 2 tennis balls
	■ 2 reaction balls
	■ Marker spots
	■ Marker drill belts
	■ Bibs
	■ Whiteboards
	■ Whiteboard pens

Key Questions and Assessment Strands
- Why do we need to move efficiently during sporting activities? (A&D; H&F; E&I)
- What do: form and mechanics; reactions; fast feet; and agility mean?

G+T Extension Work/SEN
- Vary teaching style and level of teacher intervention. Use verbal and non-verbal communication methods (whiteboards)
- Pupils to work in groups (pupil-selected)
- Q&A prompts relating to pupils' existing knowledge – draw upon pupils existing knowledge of sporting performance

Preparing a programme

A successful training programme should be periodised, varied, provide challenges, recognise individual needs and accommodate unscheduled changes. It must avoid demotivating youngsters by giving too much of the same, which may lead to compromised performances.

GUIDELINES

- Start with Dynamic Flex

- Complete explosive work and sprints early in a session

- An explosive session is followed by a light technique preparation day

- Progress from simple to complex drills

- Vary proportions of work to rest periods

- Develop strength before performing plyometrics

- Keep sessions short with the emphasis on *quality movement*

- Teach one new skill a day

- 3:2 work:rest ratio, e.g. 5 mins:2 mins

- Ensure *challenge* by increasing intensity, skill difficulty, and perfection of movement; do not simply add sets and reps

- NB: There are 4 stages to agility development; everything learned athletically occurs in stages and agility is no exception: Balance, Co-ordination, Programmed Agility, Random Agility.

Saq Training programme for a youth sports team

OVERVIEW

Session 1	Dynamic Flex	
	Mechanics	50%
	Innervation	30%
	Explosion	20%
	Warm-down	

Session 2	Dynamic Flex	
	Mechanics	45%
	Innervation	25%
	Accumulation	15%
	Explosion	15%
	Warm-down	

Session 3	Dynamic Flex	
	Accumulation	50%
	Explosion	40%
	Warm-down	

Session 4	Dynamic Flex	
	Mechanics	35%
	Innervation	25%
	Accumulation	25%
	Explosion	15%
	Warm-down	

Session 5	Dynamic Flex	
	Mechanics	30%
	Innervation	50%
	Accumulation	10%
	Explosion	10%
	Warm-down	

NB: Some flexibility may be necessary to respond to match evaluations.

Session 6	Dynamic Flex	
	Mechanics	15%
	Innervation	25%
	Accumulation	30%
	Explosion	30%
	Warm-down	

Session 7	Dynamic Flex	
	Accumulation	50%
	Explosion	50%
	Warm-down	

Session 8	Dynamic Flex	
	Innervation	35%
	Accumulation	35%
	Explosion	30%
	Warm-down	

Session 9	Dynamic Flex	
	Mechanics	30%
	Explosion	70%
	Warm-down	

Session 10	Dynamic Flex	
	Accumulation	50%
	Explosion	50%
	Warm-down	

Final two sessions to focus on applying sports-specific movements involving e.g. tackling, defensive movements, exploiting gaps, 3-step acceleration, deceleration before hit.

Possible Monitoring Procedures

■ Pre-Tests, e.g. 30-yard speed run/agility drill/accumulation circuit

■ Post programme – Tests repeats

■ Written feedback sheet from youngsters including pre-season individual self-assessments. General and position-specific

■ Video analysis of tests and playing performance in games.

The great advantage of these sessions is that they can be blended and fitted into existing schedules and situations to produce quality movement experiences to suit the needs of the youngsters under a teacher or coach's care. Flexibility is the key, and training can be matched to the experience and expertise of the teacher or coach. Further ideas based on QCA guidelines can be found in the Appendix.

CONCLUSION

It is hoped that your progress to this point in the book has filled you with inspiration and enjoyment. The use of the SAQ Youth Programme is both effective and extensive, covering all the abilities and aspirations found in youngsters. As an enthusiastic and committed parent, teacher or coach you should now be armed with a whole new toolkit of activities and practices to build on the already good work that you are doing.

If the type of youngster you are working with has not been catered for in this book do not be disappointed, as sports-specific SAQ books exist for those youngsters already specialising in developing their potential and special interests.

Framework as recommended by National Curriculum Schemes of Work

Objective – e.g. to teach youngsters how to sidestep

Method	Learning steps	SAQ training practices
Direct teaching	Introduction	Lateral run down ladder
Youngsters demonstrate or practise on their own/with others	Exploration	'Have a go' having seen it done
Youngsters solve problems	Exploration	Experiment with arm action and head up
Youngsters reflect on their own	Selection and application	Related to sidestep in sport 'head to head', linear down ladder
Youngsters lead others	Selection and application	Lateral ladder run, react to partner's movements outside ladder
	Consolidation and refinement	Lateral ladder run, move out and dodge partner
	Adaptation and extension	Develop Icky Shuffle then add turn and move when coming out of ladder
Youngsters officiate	Change of context/ environment	1 v. 1 in game + ball

PE National Curriculum

Below are examples of how the movement principles outlined in the SAQ Youth Programme are also indicated within the PE National Curriculum guidelines. Also outlined is a sample lesson using the appropriate objectives and outcomes.

The broad indicators of progression used to direct learning in the National PE Curriculum are placed under four aspects:

■ Acquiring and developing skills (AD)

■ Selecting and applying skills, tactical and compositional ideas (SA)

■ Knowledge and understanding of fitness and health (KU)

■ Evaluating and improving knowledge (Ev).

Key Aspects

Acquiring and developing skills

ATHLETIC ACTIVITIES: KEY STAGE 3–4

	Objectives	Outcomes
Y 7 / 8	To improve the consistency of sprinting, sustained running, jumping and throwing techniques, e.g. to teach the principles of acceleration	To perform a range of running, jumping and throwing skills with control, accuracy, power and sound technique
Y 9 / 10	To show precision, control and fluency in a range of chosen events, e.g. to develop the ability to sustain smooth sprinting action from 10 to 30 secs	To demonstrate good technique in all phases of a run or race

INVASION GAMES: KEY STAGE 3–4

	Objectives	Outcomes
Y 7 / 8	To improve the consistency, quality, adaptation and development of skills, e.g. to learn the importance of feints and acceleration when trying to outwit an opponent	To use an increasing range of personal techniques consistently, accurately and fluently while playing small-sided games
Y 9 / 10	To apply techniques to the game, e.g. to investigate the skills needed in a number of positions	To adapt and improvise techniques to suit different situations
Y 10 / 11	To plan and make use of advanced techniques, e.g. to refine ability to send, receive and travel with the ball	To use an increasing range of game-specific techniques with control, precision, speed and fluency

Knowledge of Fitness and Health

STRIKING AND FIELDING GAMES: KEY STAGE 3–4

	Objectives	Outcomes
Y 7 / 8	To prepare for and recover from exercise effectively and safely and know the principles used, e.g. to learn exercises that will help develop speed and reactions	To identify the principle that speed, power and quick reactions are needed to play these games well
Y 9 / 10	To know how to continue to improve personal fitness in and through games, e.g. to understand the need for flexibility and quick reactions	To explain what has to happen to become fitter for these games

KNOWLEDGE OF FITNESS AND HEALTH: KEY STAGE 3–4

	Objectives	Outcomes
Y 10 / 11	To devise, implement and monitor own fitness programmes, e.g. to understand the way that power, co-ordination and balance are affected by fitness levels	To construct an activity programme that will deliver an agreed set of targets

SAQ Youth Programme

In Year 11 youngsters should use an increasing range of game-specific techniques with control, precision, speed and fluency. They should adapt skills appropriately and effectively to meet the needs of the situation (QCA Schemes of Work). Here is an example of how these objectives and outcomes can be met by using SAQ Training as part of a lesson:

KS 4 – Y11 Hockey
Lesson 8

Area of Activity: GAMES
Topic: Explosive multidirectional movement

LESSON AIM **To develop more explosive multi directional movements so as to improve attacking play in and around the shooting circle.**

LESSON OBJECTIVES	LESSON OUTCOMES
AD – Plan for and make use of advanced techniques	Use an increasing range of game-specific techniques with control, precision, speed and fluency
SA – Adapt strategies and tactics as needed, e.g. extending the ability to anticipate and position	Use complex patterns of play
KU – Devise, implement and monitor fitness programmes appropriate for the chosen game	Design programmes to improve skills, fitness and tactics
EV – Improve analytical skills and thereby develop performance	Identify strengths and preferences in different activities and roles

Warm up – Dynamic Flex (10 mins) See sports-specific warm-up (page 4). Finish with a burst of short ladder work including backward movement outside ladder and turns at each end.

Accumulation of Potential (10 mins)

■ Accelerate, decelerate then change direction

■ Set out circuit using a ladder, followed by 4 cones, another ladder and 3 cones in a fan layout; youngster accelerates through first ladder and swerve runs around cones, decelerates through second ladder and changes direction to accelerate to one of the 3 cones as indicated by the teacher

Variation Receive ball at cone; change ladder drills.

Sets and Reps 1 set of 6 reps with walk-back recovery.

GAME (10 mins) As part of the preparatory work for a class competition as laid out in the QCA Core Task a small sided game is played applying the above practice into attacking youngsters, making appropriate forward runs to receive through passes.

Explosion (10 mins) Peel-off-and-turn work: key youngsters in each team to use Viper Belt (if one is available); youngster wearing belt loosely accelerates explosively towards a cone, moving away from the circle after 5 yards at second cone, swivels in the belt and explodes back to the circle. Other youngsters practise Let-Goes at different angles into and across the circle.

GAME (10 mins) Small-sided game, attackers versus defenders, working on explosive runs and 'cuts' into circle to set up shooting opportunities.

Warm-down Slow Dynamic Flexibility drills repeated plus static stretches.

Basic Movement Progressions

Jade, aged 9, has cerebral palsy and works on SAQ activities in her normal PE lessons together with her classmates. The lesson plan below outlines a typical lesson plan.

Ladder work	■ Linear – Dead Leg moving right/left foot forwards in each square ■ Linear – Dead Leg moving right/left foot sideways in each square ■ Linear – Single step, right foot lead, left foot steps beside, repeat ■ Single step walk, one foot in each square, alternate action ■ Linear – Single step walk, one foot in every second square to increase stride length ■ Linear – Place hurdle at start and end of ladder and in the middle ■ Linear – Place spots in different spaces to change step/stride pattern by stepping on or over ■ Place spots on outsides of ladder to encourage a step out onto spot ■ Lateral –Single step right foot lead to right ■ Single step left foot lead to left ■ Repeat but after right/left step, step forwards out of ladder space with right or left foot before continuing; repeat in other direction (variation – step back instead of forwards) ■ Place hurdles at start and end of ladder and in the middle to step over, moving sideways ■ Combination – Fold ladder into an L shape and repeat above with a change of direction ■ Fold ladder in the other direction
Spots	■ 4 spots; stand on one and reach out with one foot to tap 1 of 3 spots in front ■ Repeat, placing spots to side or in a circle ■ Use spots to determine step/stride patterns ■ Use spots to determine standing lunge patterns – walking lunges
Hurdles	■ Dead Leg over 3 hurdles, right foot/left foot lead ■ Single step-over hurdles (extend and vary spacing) ■ Square Gate of hurdles to encourage stepping over in different directions ■ 2 hurdles side by side and a spot on either side placed in the middle; step over hurdle on right, step around spot and return over other hurdle in other direction, around other spot so moving in a circle; repeat in other direction
MAKE UP OWN PATTERNS AND COMBINATIONS!	

Glossary

Ability A stable, enduring, mainly genetically defined trait that underlies skilled performance

Athleticism A natural aptitude for physical activities

Balance The ability to maintain equilibrium while in motion

Bilateral exercise An exercise using both arms or legs at the same time

Biomechanics The science that examines the internal and external factors acting on a human body and the effects produced by these forces

Complex movements Movements involving the co-ordinated working together of different functions or parts of the body

Concentric muscle contraction Contraction that involves shortening of the relevant muscle

Co-ordination The ability to perform accurate tasks, often involving the use of the senses, and a series of correlated muscular contractions affecting a range of joints and therefore relative limb and body positions

Eccentric muscle contraction Contraction that involves lengthening of the relevant muscle

Fire/Firing muscles The fast activation of specific muscle groups

Fitness The ability to carry out tasks without undue fatigue

Flexibility The range of motion through which the limbs or body parts are permitted to move

Functional movements Movements that have a specific purpose, i.e. those that relate to the specific requirements of an activity

Healthy Of strong constitution, producing well-being and vigour

Innervate To stimulate, to transmit a nervous energy to a muscle

Mechanics The technical aspects of movement

Motor skills Skills where the primary determinant of success are the movement components themselves

Neuro-muscular system The relationship between the central nervous system and the muscular system

Plyometrics Drills or exercises linking sheer strength and scope of movement to produce on explosive-reactive type of movement.

Programmed learning The systematic acquisition of new patterns of action

Proprioception Sensory information arising from the body, resulting in the sense of position and movement

Reps The number of times a task, such as a work interval or lifting of a weight, is repeated

Rhythm A sequence of regularly recurring functions

Set A group of repetitions

Simple movements A movement involving a small number of joints or muscles where co-ordination among limbs is minimized

Skill A capability to bring about an end result with maximum certainty and minimum energy and time

Strategies Overall plans for success

Strength The force that a muscle or muscle group can exert against a resistance

Tactics Detailed patterns of movement

Timing The process of regulating an action to produce the best effect

Training An exercise programme to develop an athlete for a particular event and/or to increase skill of performance and energy capacities

Velocity Speed or rate of movement

BIBLIOGRAPHY AND REFERENCES

In the same series:

Pearson, A.E. (2001), *SAQ Rugby*, A&C Black, London.

Pearson, A.E. (2001), *SAQ Soccer*, A&C Black, London.

Pearson, A.E. (2003), *SAQ Women's Soccer*, A&C Black, London.

Pearson, A.E. and Naylor, S. (2003), *SAQ Hockey*, A&C Black, London.

Pearson, A.E. (2004), *Dynamic Flexibility*, A&C Black, London.

Pearson, A.E. (2003), *Fit 4 Work*, A&C Black, London.

Bailey, Richard and Macfadyen, Tony (2000), *Teaching Physical Education 5–11*, pp. 77–80. Continuum: London.

Bailey, R. and Morley, D. (2003), 'Using Dynamic Assessment to Identify Potential Talent in Physical Education Incorporating a SAQ Programme' (available from SAQ International/Centre for Physical Education, Leeds Met Carnegie University)

Bennett, S. (1999), *t-and-f: New muscle research findings-muscle symposium*. AIS: Canberra, Australia.

Bompa Tudor, O. (2000), *Total Training for Young Champions*, Human Kinetics: New York.

Buroker, K.C., and Schwane, J.A. (1989), Does post exercise stretching alleviate DOMS. *Physician and Sportsmedicine*, 17 (6): 65–83.

De Vries, H. (1986), *Physiology of Exercise – For Physical Education and Athletics*, pp. 462–72, 474–87, 482–8. Wm.C. Brown: Dubuque, IA.

Enoka, R.M. (1994), *Neuromechanical Basis of Kinesiology*. Human Kinetics: New York.

Fowles, J.R., Sale, D.G., and MacDougall, J.D. (2000) 'Reduced strength after passive stretch of the human plantarflexors', *Journal of Applied Physiology*, 89: 1179–88.

Gallahue, David L. and Cleland Donnelly, Frances, (2003), *Developmental Physical Education for all Youngsters*, p 54. Human Kinetics: New York.

Gleim, G.W and McHugh, M.P. (1997), 'Flexibility and its effects on sports injury and performance', *Sports Medicine* 24 (5): 289–99.

Herbert, R.D., and Gabriel, M.G. (2002), 'Effects of stretching before and after exercising on muscle soreness and risk of injury: A systematic review,' *British Medical Journal*, 325: 468.

Moscov, J.G. (1993). *Static ROM, Leg Power and Strength as Predictors of Dynamic ROM in Female Ballet Dancers*. Microform Publications: University of Oregon, Eugene.

Pope, R.P., Herbert, R.D., and Kirwan, J.D. (2000), 'A randomised trial of pre-exercise stretching for the prevention of lower limb injury', *Medicine and Science in Sports and Exercise*, 32: 271–7.

Portwood, Madeleine (2000), *Developmental Dyspraxia, Identification and Intervention A Manual for Parents and Professionals*. David Fulton: London.

Portwood, Madeleine (2003), Dyslexia and Physical Education, pp. 7–9. David Fulton: London.

Qualifications and Curriculum Authority (QCA) *Physical Education Schemes of Work* – www.qca.org.uk

Rosenbaum, D., and Hennig, E.M. (1995), 'The influence of stretching and warm-up exercises on Achilles tendon reflex activity', *Journal of Sports Sciences*, 13: 481–90.

Schilling, B.K., and Stone, M.H. (2000), '"Stretching": acute effects on strength and performance', *Strength and Conditioning Journal*, 22 (1): 44–7.

Shrier, I. (1999), 'Stretching before exercise does not reduce the risk of local muscle injury: a critical review of the clinical and basic science literature', *Clinical Journal of Sports Medicine*, 9: 221–7.

Smith, L.L., Brunetz, M.H., Cheiner, T.C., McCammon, M.R., Houmard, J.A., Franklin, M.E., and Israel, R.G. (1993), 'The effects of static and ballistic stretching on DOMS and Creatin Kinase', *Research Quarterly for Exercise and Sport*, 64 (1): 103–7.

Smythe, R. (1994), *Journal of Training and Conditioning*.

INDEX OF DRILLS

LIBRARY, UNIVERSITY OF CHESTER